Onésimo Fernández Rubio

# AT SUNSET

# AT SUNSET

Summary of a life partially dedicated to psychiatric care

Onésimo Fernández Rubio

Onésimo Fernández Rubio



ISBN: 978-8469753965

THANKS TO

Anunciata Baquer Masgrau, colleague, friend and invaluable adviser.

Dionisio González de Andrés, friend and supervisor of these pages.

Cover Design
María Collado Bailo

DEDICATION

Maria Luisa left early, hardly knowing us. Recently, our beloved brother, Josemari, has also gone. Perhaps he is busy making ice cream, in the sky, so that when we arrive we will not feel nostalgic for those delicious ice creams which, together with Paca and Onésimo, prepared at the Casino of our beloved Valencia de Don Juán (Coyanza).

In your indelible memory, your brothers dedicate you these lines, which belong to everyone equally, and also to you.

To the memory of our loved companions: Tomy and Daf, as well.

# INDEX

# AL ATARDECER

# FOREWORD

"This is a book without any prevention."

This is the first thought that came to my mind after I finished reading it.

Dr. Fernández Rubio presents a way of looking at psychiatry from a different perspective than how "official" psychiatry does. Based on the experience of many years of work, the human mind goes from the birth to the last measures of life in a clear and concise way and without any complexes. He does not care if his opinions are well received by the academic world or not; are their opinions, basically based on psychoanalysis, and expresses them in a way that even the uninitiated in this matter can understand.

The reader who enters in this book will find the reason for human suffering, the reasons why we act in some ways and not in others, the differences between freedom and free will and an endless number of issues that everyone, sooner or later, we ask ourselves when things "do not go" as we wish.

I encourage the reader to sit comfortably, with relaxing background music, and go into the exciting world of the psyche, of the soul, without haste and, without any kind of taboo, meditate on what he is reading. It is not an easy book, it is dense, hence my recommendation to read it slowly, to meditate on it. Whether you agree with the theories contained in these pages or not, you will not remain indifferent.

Dr. Enrique Cremades Martín

# 1. PREAMBLE

As when on the beaches, the first rains of September indicate to the vacationers that the holidays are about to end, these lines also warn me that my wandering through the fields of Psychiatry is touching its end. From now on, what has happened will remain in the memory and only from that corner can be evoked as a summary, as when the pages of a book have been passed and mental content is reviewed.

The silence is taking possession of the hubbub and the loneliness dominates the crowded places that gradually become deserted. The bustle of days ago is gone, and the stillness takes over the once lively places, while a nostalgic autumn mist descends over the now desolate spaces.

As I say, of the past only the memory will remain and, recorded in it, the most representative passages that, as a cairn, will serve for its evocation. Finally, from everything only will remain the impalpable feeling of when there is no possibility of return. It is the same feeling that today encourages me to write this summary, the extract of my entire professional life. At the final stretch of my path, already visible the goal, these pages that are the sediment of my entire journey through the path of Psychiatry, have no other purpose than to be a mere personal relief. Or, at most, that of a testimony: the mine.

As the pilgrim, who sees the end of the journey, free from the burden of the hesitations of the departure, has installed in me a perspective of adventure begun years ago. Many of the aspirations, outside the strict competence of the psychiatric profession, have been detached with each stride. Thus, in my case, lightened by the weight of the conventions and requirements of everyday life, it is possible for me to show the experience without the impurities and hindrances that impose, both the submission to established postulates and the servitude of the inevitable ambitions of the years of youth.

And, since this exposition is not intended to rise above other "truths", nor does it aspire to be a springboard for the attainment of notoriety or advantage, it may easily be subject to the purpose of being a mere transcription of my intimate conversations. With this, I put myself in the shelter of criticism, while being freed of justifications. Because, pretending nothing, beyond a meager release, no loss I have to fear. This is, fortunately, my position.

It is a pity that the nature of this matter, and my clumsiness too, prevent a less categorical exposition, more attached to the lyricism that, despite the drama, have the passages of the lives on which this writing rests, but this is a limitation that does not I can avoid.

On the other hand, the following lines continue the ideas expressed in my previous publication, "The Sickness of Life", although today purified and strengthened by the passage of the days.

For convenience, I omit to cite the different authors to whom, directly or indirectly, more than to myself, the opinions expressed belong, although I recognize me in them from the dawn of my life, for I think that I have been revolving around the same notion of the existence, already present in my earliest memories, just as the donkey revolves around the waterwheel, even though in its fantasy it creates free jogging for the green meadows. Thus, stating that I owe everything, I don't need to fulfil the laborious task of saturating the pages of calls. In addition, what happens here is the same as when we underline the sentences or paragraphs of a reading that, believing to discover something new, we only highlights what had already been borrowed by intuition, but exposed in a more clear and original.

Besides, since the purpose of this paper is to refer to what has been left over during my professional practice, it would not be appropriate to refer, at each point, to the author to whom this or that idea might be due. But, in addition, it is not only isolated ideas that will find accommodation here; on the contrary, it is a global and personal conception of psychiatric discipline, away from technicalities and attached to everyday existence, to life itself.

Come to this point, I have serious doubts about that the people being able to learn guidelines for better living or, in any case, we should do so with little effectiveness, so that we could very well spend the days of existence turning around the same ideas that were configured at the same moment of opening our eyes and that, consequently, the days of our lives would be consummated in the mere consolidation of those early impressions.

Well, under these conditions I write these pages, but not because I think it will bring something new or beneficial, not; simply, pushed by the same expressive need that leads us to externalize the contents of the soul.

## 2. INTRODUCTION

These pages are intended to show the sediment of a life occupied in the exercise of Psychiatry, and they want to carry out with the same mood with which the pilgrim faces the conclusion of his path, who at the end of his adventure, believes to have a particular Impression about the meaning of the trip, something like a sediment, compendium of all the sensations and experiences that make up our particular sense of existence, despite knowing that it is something unfathomable and indefinable.

If possible any choice, few doubts I might have about the motive that drove me towards the psychiatric profession, which must have been the curiosity to find an explanation about the meaning of our stay in life and the meaning of the variety of behaviours , Sometimes paradoxical: this, I believe, is the incentive that drives this company.

If one thinks logically, it is surprising that, at the height of humanity's current development, there are those still living in the obsession to defend genetic, chemical and neurological causes, in blatant omission of emotional factors, to know the sources of spiritual suffering. And, I say it is surprising because, to my understanding, the explanations about spiritual discomfort are clear and unobjectionable, without having to leave the psychological sphere. In addition, it seems sterile to resort to uncertain causes that the future could confirm, or not, when in our hands we have simple and sufficient explanations.

I say to be surprised by these attitudes, although, on the other hand, it is unavoidable to try to understand them, because the pressing interests of subsistence displaced, by inopportune, those of greater transcendence and, because life runs between narrow margins that hardly allow daring.

Going back on these steps, I have the impression that we are still slaves of prejudices such as those who dogmatize that only those who pass the mathematical proof can be admitted as truths, as if there were no other certainties outside of them. In my previous publication II dedicated some comment about "the scientific", so that I will not repeat it. I will only comment that there are necessarily facts that are true in themselves without necessity of their mathematical demonstration. Such is the case of grief, joy, tenderness, need, contrariety, day and night and endless happenings of existence. Descartes came to the assurance of existing by thinking; In the same way he could reach the same conclusion by appealing to feeling, suffering, joy or tears.

The obstinacy in seeking causes outside the psychological realm is as foolish a conduct as it would be that of one who, lost in the desert, scorned the water of a rickety spring waiting to stumble upon an oasis.

And I say this because to all the congresses, forums and meetings, I attended, all the interventions, all, ended with the same pretentious sentence: "Not today, but in the short future it is expected that this path will lead us to the solution. A path has been initiated that will lead to the achievement of the proposed goal". And all this always referred to a promising new drug, although common sense warns us that a drug has to be certainly miraculous to meet the demand for as many requests as they are aroused in any spiritual manifestation.

The stubbornness of reality has postponed, as it could not be otherwise, the confirmation of such foolish hopes, while "scientific" meetings continue their course amid empty lectures and masterful lessons, establishing a clear dissociation between the exercise of everyday life of the specialty - which must take place in the privacy of the cabinet - and the bombasticness of academic discourses; between real life and the life of university chairs.

If I were to find myself at the beginning of the exercise of the profession, with vanity still intact and ambition unchecked, it would surely work in the classical way: I would try to define the concepts that have been the framework of the psychiatric specialty (illness, symptom, etiology, etc.), I would try, later. A classification of my own and proceed in the same way with the remaining elements (treatment, prognosis, etc.)

until reaching the end. But, I repeat, it does not aspire to be an original treaty but rather the equivalent of what, referred to culture, was defined by the author of relativity, Albert Einstein, as "what remains of sediment after forgetting all the memorized", but applied to the sphere of Psychiatry.

As in any exposition, however objective it may be, the biographical components play an important role, and so in my case the particular conditions of my life have led me along the path of simplicity, without this word having a pejorative connotation; It is not good or bad in itself, it simply is. Because, exercising a moral judgment about the facts would commit the same folly as the one who, studying the literary currents of "Conceptismo" (Literary school that emphasizes the value of the concept over that of the form) and the "Culteranismo" (the opposite school), to give an example, end up affirming the superiority of one over the other -both being at the service of expression literary-, will forget to highlight the particularities of each one of them.

Incidentally, if I had been living in the midst of these currents, I would surely be closer to the conceptual school.

Digressions aside, what I want to make clear is that all my education has led me to simplicity, to synthesis, to pay preferential attention to the bottom rather than the form. From my examinations of faculty I remember that, for the fulfillment of the same task that other colleagues needed ten or more pages, I was enough with one; And counting on knowing the answers. This inclination toward the simple is a characteristic that has accompanied me throughout all my life.

Going back on the steps, I believe that no one can proclaim sensibly not to understand of Psychiatry, as no one can claim to have no notion about justice, because both, unlike other well-delimited technical specialties, such as computer science, deal with the universal interests of existence and about them, whether they want it or not, we all inevitably have our own opinion. And what could psychiatry do if it were not the facts of life itself and also the particular way in which the circumstances shape the form of existence of each? The psychiatric discipline can not deal with any other matter than the orderly reconstruction, step by step, of the way in which biographical accidents have been shaping the genuine way of being the person in the world, just as the channel leads the waters of the river, conditioning his course.

Before continuing, I think it is convenient to make a distinction between the terms "being" and "to be in the world", between essence and circumstance. A person can "to be in the world" as a cabinetmaker, to set an example, but not "being" a cabinetmaker. For in this example, "being in the world" as a cabinetmaker is the circumstance, the accident of which "being" is its own essence.

Basically, the person is a creature forced to adapt to the environment. Well, The Psychiatry studies the antecedents and circumstances that explain the particular way of his "being in the world". For if there is a characteristic that properly belongs to being, is that of plasticity, a property derived, in turn, from helplessness and necessity. First, the child must be mouldable to traverse the birth channel. And this demand that nature presents in the biological plane requires it, equally, for the spiritual sphere.

The child appears in life provided with the same instinctive flow destined, fundamentally, to its approach to pleasure and the flight from the suffering. The position of "being in the world" is determined by its interaction with the environmental conditions to which, full of necessity as he arrives, must necessarily be adapted, in the same way that the helmsman is forced to, temporarily, give part of the course to overcome currents and storms Impossible to cope with. Later, and as far as possible, throughout the course of life the person will try to accommodate the world at his convenience, although by then he will have sculpted the features that will determine his particular way of "being in the world".

Observing the behaviour of the child, we intuit that the same instinctive flow -in my opinion constant for everybody-, necessarily in conflict with the impositions of the caregivers and the requirements of coexistence, to which he has to pay a fee. For if we were all allowed to evolve spontaneously, without hindrance -an impossible thing- we would exhibit, with few variations, identical behaviours.

The fears of the caretakers, or the risks of the environment, make the child to conform to their requirements, thus initiating the construction of their particular way of being, having to deliver in this process part of what would have been their spontaneous evolution. The sequence of this interminable cession, similar to what happens when we cross a path of brambles in which the strips of the dress remain, describes the gradual loss of the signs of individual identity, which in extremely unfavourable circumstances turn the person into a mere representative of others' aspirations. In other words, environmental impositions can explain later how a person can be stripped of his being, to a greater or lesser degree, and become the seat of aspirations of others, and these assignments may even end in the annihilation of one's being. When this unfortunate outcome takes place, the person contemplates the discourse of the days of his existence, without being allowed to intervene in his own adventure, never to occupy "his position", without reaching the goal of being "himself/herself" or, which is equal, taking care of the benefit of others. In a nutshell: living in alienation.

This is the real existential conflict and its reconstruction, step by step, is the true task of the psychiatric discipline.

From the above, I understand that Psychiatry is a discipline that deals with the study, in voluntary collaboration with the applicant, of the gradual incidence of obstacles in personal development, which will explain, in turn, the greater or lesser detention of the process -always to culminate- which leads to the establishment of the person in the world as being "herself", a work which, incidentally, has close similarity to that of the archaeologist.

This statement departs from the classic definitions that understand psychiatry as the discipline in charge of the care of so-called mental illnesses. For the term illness, which comes from bodily medicine, cannot be applied to psychiatric discipline without the necessary correction, otherwise one can fall into the vice derived from its original meaning, from the "different," in addition to the moral nuance that the term "disease" has been acquiring throughout the evolution of Psychiatry.

The Psychiatric discipline is a recent addition to traditional medicine, essentially materialistic. The improving of the living conditions of modern society has brought new demands and, the same than other medical disciplines, such as plastic surgery, to put an example that attends new needs different than the ancient medicine in which the maintenance of life was the main objective. It is for this reason that the term disease, thus taken, does not acquire a full meaning without proper purifications for its actualization and use in spiritual medicine. On the other hand, what significance would it have, in Psychiatry, to speak of disease when in this term biographical aspects are not included?

It seems to me more adjusted to reality to speak of suffering. For, although biographical considerations may be understood to be relatively secondary to the understanding of a physical illness, as in the case of an infection, to put an example, this is not the case when it is the understanding of something that presents itself with enigmatic traits, as it is the case of a panic attack, apparently unchained by the fact of not being in the seat near the exit of the projection room. The word disease has a certain degree of partiality, of affecting limited bodily areas, as in fractures, for example. The term suffering, however, affects the person as a whole and has to do with the whole set of avatars of his existence. If to this difference is added the fact that, even in present times, the spiritual suffering is associated an inappropriate and negative moral burden and a sense of responsibility, if not the guilt, we will understand better the reason for the need for differentiation between both terms.

In both forms, the person undergoes, passively, its effects without any intervention in its causation. In nothing the essence of the person is affected, only in his circumstance. Neither sickness nor suffering are inherent to the "being" but are part of their "being in the world", so that a law can be established which, on the spiritual plane, could be stated as follows: "under similar conditions, all persons would exhibit identical manifestations"

Another crazy imitation of classical medicine is the attempt of classification of mental manifestations. In this respect, it will suffice to comment that all the efforts aimed at typecasting, such as those carried out by the authors of the CIE and DSM manuals, are doomed to failure. The exuberant expressiveness of the person escapes any attempt to be inventoried, much less valued. This difficulty explains his incessant updates, in an idle effort that only finds some kind of justification in the elaboration of protocols destined to the "defensive medicine".

I'll explain. The extension of medical care to the whole population -a fact that is undoubtedly a formidable social achievement - has, however, serious drawbacks, particularly with regard to psychiatric care, since it tends to generalize what is of nature Individual, person to person. In outpatients, for example, psychiatric care follows a protocol that begins with the exposition of the reason for the consultation, and the corresponding biographical references, to an interposed person. Only after this filter is passed, the client is received by the psychiatrist; thus, he's forced to "undress" twice before two unknown people. It is clear that this nonsense has to obey interests outside the own assistance, such as the promotion of various health care, a task enthusiastically cheered by the unions in this ever-pending revolution. You can vaccinate in group, for example, but there are certain types of care that have to be personalized. Psychiatric care is one of them.

The present times, characterized by a greater demand and responsibility in the medical exercise, bring with them, a flow of complaints, an aspect which, although it has advantages, also, as it happens with the "nocturnal attack" of the teachings of military tactics, has also drawbacks. As a consequence, appears the asepsis, the coldness and the suspicion, in the physician-patient relationships, and with them, the birth of the protocols of action, a guideline whose follow-up puts the professional in the shelter of possible claims, although this action not always be the most convenient.

Two antecedents explain the current situation: on the one hand, the pride of the medical collective, addict to appearing in the public media proclaiming the advances of therapeutics, which, in turn, has led to the extension of the belief that death is a medical failure and on the other, the disorientation of judges and magistrates who very often transgress the framework of their representation to invade the fields of Psychology, imposing millionaires sanctions. The result of all this is the defensive attitude of the medical action as well as the indiscriminate and exhaustive use of proofs, no matter if indicated or not, in order to be protected by the protocol.

Going back to the section in which were highlighted the differences between the medicine of the body and that of the spirit, it will be accepted that, for the latter as opposed to the practical spirit prevailing in the first, everything that belongs to the realm of fantasy will have the higher interest. It seems incredible that opinions are still held that defend the uselessness of a phenomenon, and what, for a scientific mind is even more surprising, is that there may be manifestations that do not participate with the rest of what constitutes the fact of the individual life and with the individual himself. Particularly, the psychiatric practice suffers, probably to a greater extent than any other specialty, of this defect; hence the foolish effort to waste the energies trying to eradicate the symptoms, which are nothing more but the appearances of a more hidden reality. This also explains the failure of successive plans for reforming psychiatric care, more driven by electoral and aesthetic aspirations than dictated by the knowledge and understanding.

Psychiatry, as well as other branches of knowledge, such as botany, to give an example, has followed the same evolutionary steps: starting from the description of what is observed and finding similarities that make possible the grouping in families, until finding a common nexus to all. It is understood that the first phase -the descriptive one-, in the absence of another understanding, be exhausted in hollow erudition based on the unfounded belief that by the fact of naming something one enters into the possession of his knowledge. In this we hardly get rid from the innate human propensity to the magical and the miraculous spirit, which leads to the belief of dominating something by the mere fact of having adjudicated a name. This is the artistic stage, that of the elaborate clinical accounts, of the prolific reports: the literary stage, in short. This moment corresponds the Psychiatry I met in the chairs and in the congresses. To such a lack of understanding belongs the blind application of successive remedies (shock therapies and the administration of the whole range of psychotropic drugs), as well as the never-ending hope of finding the definitive solution in a miraculous preparation.

The medicine is probably the discipline in which with more frequency it gets confused the fact that knowing a phenomenon is similar of having baptized it. This irrational proceeding is complemented by the widespread custom of applying the irrefutable "scientifically proven" sentence when no objection is to be admitted. Perhaps this deception is the explanation of why medicine has collected many of the former churchgoers, and one of the two great vices with which the understanding stumbles. In the same sense, the profuse use of acronyms, imitations of the magical words of shamans and religious officiants, has the intention of, in addition to persuading the others of the possession of a debatable knowledge, to put to that one that manifests it, under the protection against possible claims.

With the same intentionality, care protocols have been instituted, a rigorous of an inappropriate extension of surgical asepsis to the rest of the medical profession, which in reality constitute veritable shelters against the judicial claims.

As already happened in botany, here too, as the knowledge of functions progresses, the description becomes less important. Something similar to what happened in my time as a student of anatomy when two chairs, governed by two people with almost opposite sensibilities: one inclined to the meticulous description of anatomical accidents and another more interested in the function of the muscles that were anchored there. Thus, in Psychiatry, the more one advances in knowledge, the more unanimously one accepts that exists a symptom par excellence, the anguish, from which all others emerge.

Incidentally I will point out that anguish, described as a disease by eminent colleagues, is nothing more than the medium in which life develops itself, the air we breathe; It is not any disease. In this issue, as in so many others as tuberculosis, ringworm, rickets, etc., will be the times with their technological advances - and not so much the progress of medicine itself- that will determine their decline.

The repetition leads to the simplification of steps that at first appeared so convoluted that, in my thinking of then, they were only within the reach of privileged minds and that, in the end, many of them turned out to be just a fools and charlatans. Such is the way that leads to the acquisition of what has always been called "to have office". Thus, the exercise of Psychiatry has brought me to a point where what once seemed complex and reserved for exceptional characters, shows me simple, clear, diaphanous.

Today I contemplate things full of simplicity and it is by virtue of this that I invite the reader, if any, to follow, step by step, the natural course of what is the exercise of this specialty, instead of beginning with the description of the entities and the like. To do this, let us follow the path of someone who comes to the consultation; the expectations that lead there, of what often finds there and the conditions that surround it.

It seems artificial to me the distinction between Psychology and Psychiatry since both would be meaningless if they deviated from the study of the psyche, the soul.

# 3. THE PSYCHIATRIC CONSULTATION

The psychiatric practice begins at the moment of the consultation and this, like the other consultations, has a well defined components: the reason itself, which is the story; the person who expresses it, the client; and who receives it, the psychiatrist.

Before these three elements come into contact, it would seem unnecessary to add that everything that takes place between the four walls of the cabinet must be surrounded by an atmosphere in line with confidentiality and freedom. The socialization of health care unfortunately makes that these requirements are not met.

The spiritual suffering can be expressed through its very different manifestations, such as dizziness (people who can't travel sitting in the contrary sense of movement on buses), restlessness, phobia, obsession, depression, delirium and hallucination, among others, besides of a varied sample of body expressions. Through these manifestations, of the so called symptoms, the spiritual suffering is expressed. His verbalization is the link between client and doctor.

The object of the consultation is materialized in the patient's story and is, in essence, the expression of the symptom which, as has been said, can be shown through very varied appearances, all of them advertisers of a suffering whose cause is not directly understandable through the use of reason, but is hidden in the domains of the so-called unconscious. In Psychiatry, unlike what happens in organic medicine, the symptoms (washing hands repeatedly without being able to avoid it, for example), impose themselves in a fatal and incomprehensible way for those who suffer them, causing, besides their uneasiness, the impotence for being slave of such an absurd ritual. For how understand that being clean is not possible to avoid washing them, again and again, in spite being clean? This enigmatic and imperious character is what justifies the presence of the psychiatrist, who has the role of unravelling its meaning.

With respect to the symptom it is convenient to make some precisions. First, do not confuse the terms cause and symptom. Symptom, as I say, is the way to manifest an intimate happening, something similar to what happens with smoke and fire. Therefore, it is not only a nuisance; it is the simplified manifestation of a complex happening that concerns the entire life of the individual. The verbal exposition of the symptom expresses only the appearance of the conflict.

But it is also that the symptom is not something trivial, it is a reservoir of potential energy that, if sequestered, can't enter into the general stream and to pass the disposition of the individual, who thus depletes his capacity to manage life. Therefore, it is not something that, if it were viable, it would be appropriate to eliminate, because this would amputate many of the possibilities of the sufferer. This energy, subjected to the powerful processes of repression, can find discharge, besides to the creation of symptoms psychic, in the creation of physical alterations through the process known as somatisation.

The advance of physical science, the precursor of today's prodigious instruments of physical exploration, is, in a great way, the cause of the conceit of the organic medicine and its contempt for the aforementioned process of transformation of psychic conflicts into somatic alterations.

The inappropriate pharmacological orientation of Psychiatry also explains the mistakes that occur in this field, probably more pronounced than in any other and that are evident in the hospital units for the treatment of anorexia -true torture enclosures-, in the crazy units for the attention of the drug addition, in the abuse of pharmacological prescriptions, in the inappropriate use of behavioral guidance, in the misguided units of attention to the so-called Alzheimer's disease, in the creation of insomniac units of sleep, in the painful units of pain and in the endless absurdities.

The use of psychological knowledge in the recruitment of soldiers in the Second World War was already an aberrant one, because nothing is more contrary to psychological assistance than the application of its knowledge for the purposes other than the identification of obstacles that prevent the person to reach the goal of being "himself". But it seems that in this, as in many other activities, it follows the police orientation such as when they oblige to urinate to the patient in the presence of "medical commissars" who do not even have intention to understand the phenomena are in front of their observation.

In this confusion, the widespread "doctrine of contagion" also plays a prominent role. The same isolation technique, pertinent in dealing with infectious diseases in which there is a risk of exposure to the pathogenic focus, has been transferred, without criticism, to the psychological world, made particularly evident in the campaign against the anorexia to the point of prohibiting the parade to models that do not reach a certain weight. In the background beats unscathed the conviction of the irresistible seduction that has the temptation of sin, in this case in the form of food, surprising circumstance for all those who knew times of poverty and hunger.

Another of the mistakes of Psychiatry, in its practical aspect, is to consider the symptom as an isolated fact, futile, capable of being judged and corrected, as if it were a whim or a debauched behaviour. No attempt to understand that the symptoms could be the consequence of certain causes and that the diversity of their presentations had no other purpose than to be signs of help that the being throws outside in its effort not to perish.

Anguish is the fundamental symptom from which all others derive. The word comes from Latin and means narrowness, narrowing, difficulty, and speaks of an unconscious conflict that always has as meaning the fear, not to die physically, but to perish as being.

Let us return to the different steps that take place in the psychiatric consultation. In reference to the narrative it is not idle to notice that the client's narrative is, by definition, truthful and corresponds to the accumulation of experiences and personal interpretations, so that it can't be doubted, but must be received as it comes from his lips. The psychiatrist should not judge about its authenticity, but the investigation of its meaning. The story is, therefore, unquestionable.

One could argue that the person, thus presenting things, could have disfigured, deformed or misinterpreted. But does it prevent the archaeologist from fulfilling his task that the passage of time has been able to modify the remains of his investigation? Otherwise, what to do, if so? Who is the object of attention: the person who goes to the cabinet or, on the contrary, the world that believes to perceive with greater clarity what the patient has lived and that constitutes his reality? The absence of a correct approach makes this obvious truth lend itself to being an artificial disjunction, because what the client refers is a product of their experiences and the interpretation of them. In its acceptance there can be no objection. The opposite would be so much as to tell him that he should not interpret things as he does, which would lead us to consider him incapable. There is no more cruel form of rejection that the questioning the story.

Therefore, the inexcusable requirement for the establishment of a therapeutic relationship is the acceptance of the narrative as it is referred and that contains real facts in all senses whose authenticity is unquestioned. The psychiatrist is a researcher, not a policeman. Besides, enough cops and trials are hidden behind the symptoms of those who come to the consulting room to add more burden to the work started in their remote times. The acceptance of the story, as it comes from the lips of the client, is also based on the unquestionable reality that what he expresses are experiences that he suffers impotent and to which he reacts with the weapons that life has provided. Therefore, the story is authentic in itself. The psychiatrist's mission is to unravel the hidden plot behind him, so he could hardly do so if he starts from the suspicion. Questioning the data is as much as labelling the person as a phony or what is the same: to become a judge.

Not even in the case of the person suffering from delusional ideation, that reacts to imaginary stimuli, this statement would lose validity, because the delusional content certainly refers to past experiences. The psychiatrist's job is to find the missing links that would make sense of what apparently seem not to have it.

The work of the psychiatrist is simple: it consists on ordering a story only seemingly incoherent; something like reshaping a puzzle to a congruent figure or unravelling a tangled ball.

But first and foremost, the psychiatrist must allow to anyone who speaks to him, to speak. It seems incredible, that this observation has to be made! But that is because the fact of having received a degree does not exempt the graduate from having to listen to the client's story, nor does he place him in a position of wisdom such that he has nothing to learn from his story, he would not even have to listen to it.

On the other hand, the framework in which the consultation takes place requires particular conditions. In the first place, it must be taken for granted that the person comes freely and not driven by his ascendants. Voluntariness is here, as in life in general, unavoidable requirement. This, which is common sense, does not seem so evident in the world of psychiatric care in which it may be that the professional is coerced by the urgency of a situation, as in family fears of the threat of Suicide of one of its members, for example.

Privacy is another indispensable element. The socializing disposition of psychiatric care in the public system which, among other nonsense, imposes the narrative on the nurse, as a prerequisite for the interview with the psychiatrist, violates the principle of privacy, the maintenance of professional secrecy and common sense.

This observation would be unnecessary by the mere fact that the psychiatrist was in possession of the necessary empathy, of this capacity to put himself in the place of the "other" or, simply, of the possibility of following the evangelical recommendation: "do with the others as you would like the others do with you". But the ability to be reflected in the neighbour is not acquired in the faculty. This idolized "scientism" has made us forget that, first of all, we are people and as such we can contemplate ourselves in the mirror of others. For the exercise of Psychiatry, the absence of these gifts is particularly harmful.

In reference to the psychiatric task it is necessary to distinguish two attitudes that involve the same numbers of models of approach to the symptom: on the one hand, those who understand that their function is to unravel the meaning hidden behind it and another, that of those who are moved by the sole purpose of its eradication. Something similar to what happens in the world of political leaders in which some have the ultimate goal of triumph in elections and others that contemplate the rise to power as the only means to develop ideas for the common welfare.

Theoretically it could be accepted the validity of these two orientations of not being because it is impossible the release of the symptom if it is not through its enlightenment since this one is but the expression of a suffering that manifests itself of form disfigured, crazy if it is wanted. If the symptom is, as has been said, the equivalent of the smoke that announces to the fire, the fireman would act erroneously directing the flow of water towards it. In the same desman would incur the psychiatrist using the efforts in its impossible eradication; I say impossible because, even if it were possible to move it to another form of manifestation, at the end it would be nothing more than a useless maneuver, such as the one used by the ostrich who, hiding his head, thinks that has mocked of his persecutor. Because, I repeat, the symptom is the succinct manifestation of a larger event.

In spite of the century that has passed since Freud's publications, it is surprising that the person is still viewed as an object for description, as one could do with the branches of a tree, different each of them, without repairing the common start of the same trunk and the same roots. In this way you can spend hours in the detailed description without this translating into any knowledge. To this fragmentary form of observation may be due to the use of the term "reification", the transformation of the complex into something elementary and extraneous.

Who asks for the consultation is because he is the bearer of an incomprehensible suffering, an enigma that causes him a grief that he does not understand and that, deposited in competent hands, hopes to be clarified. This will seem a simple thing, but it will not be seen that way if we notice the frequent use of psychological tests, which is a way of torpedoing communication.

The role of Psychiatry is similar to that of archaeology: it is a research work, which starts from a few clues -the patient's story- and tries to link missing links in the chain of the past so that it acquires a complete sense. It must, therefore, be a reconstruction effort.

In the performance of psychiatric care, unlike what is required in other more technician activities, such as computer science, personal characteristics are decisive. The technique occupies here a very secondary place. In the exercise of any other profession the results are practically identical for a varied group of people, given that the primordial, the way of proceeding, is basically the same. But in Psychiatry, where technical support is scarce and so easy is the interference of subjective opinions, it is where personal characteristics are determinant.

The sympathy aroused by commiseration is appropriate for compassionate accompaniment, but in Psychology true sympathy is the result of understanding. Therefore, and regardless of any other consideration, the story moves us and promptly provokes our adhesion and this is because we simply understand their situation. On the contrary, those who do not reach this explanation, those who do not enjoy that capacity, will not be able to experience that sympathy, their work will become tedious and soon they will become indisposed with the client and will end up confronting, even mocking about their "rarities."

A prior warning: how many opinions are to be expressed don't constitute at all criticism or disparagement towards the behaviours or opinions of their promoters, since, as I have noticed, no one is to judge them. They would, on the contrary, be samples by which I try to highlight the passion and confusion that come together in this discipline. I would also like to make it clear that, for me, the true therapeutic procedure begins with the research method derived from the studies of Sigmund Freud (1856-1939), with Psychoanalysis. Although in the nature no event can be studied isolated from de others, it can be said that the appearance of Freud's work marks a before and after in psychiatric discipline, a separation between merely descriptive and deductive Psychiatry, Psychoanalysis is, essentially a research method. His contribution inaugurates a new psychiatric era, presided over by the belief that there can be coherence in the seemingly absurd, rationality in the outwardly unreasonable. It is, in the field of Psychology, the first scientific movement tending to find the connections between causes and effects. Freud initiated not only a therapeutic procedure but the "therapeutic procedure itself."

Freud met himself with brilliant collaborators, many of whom remained loyal to the founder. Others, as always happens in the formation of groups and more when the founder is of an extraordinary category, left the group due, apparently, to theoretical discrepancies. Such were the cases of Carl Jung and Alfred Adler who, by pretext of doctrinal divergences, forgot the sources of their initiations and incapable of the logical recognition, they put themselves openly before the teacher. The ruthless passage of time has practically cornered them in the oblivion.

Today, there are still murky contradictions around the figure of Freud. For example the interview, published in a weekly national newspaper, to one of our most esteemed representatives of the psychiatric world who tells that: "reading Freud's work changed my life", adding in the next paragraph that "Psychoanalysis is very useful for healthy people, for to know the inner world and thus broaden their horizons, but as a therapeutic method is useless". When he recalls his childhood and remembers the role of the parents and their forecasts about his future, he adds: "I felt orphaned but knowing it, heals". Here is a sample of the incoherence in which one is incurred when has oneself as different from the others.

Obviously, those who care about others will benefit from the ability not to mix their ideological, political, religious and moral positions in the company. Particularly, they will enjoy being free of those paranoid positions, so frequent among so-called "political scientists", who contemplate the world ruled by a person, or association of beings, with malicious purposes, as often happens. "Wise" historians who believe they are in possession of the key that would have saved humanity from all the evils it has been suffering, still suffer and will surely suffer in the future. But the history of humanity is too complex for any expert to have such a degree of penetration.

Excessive material ambition is another pernicious travelling companion, as well as the urgency to find immediate connections between causes and effects; a pretension as absurd as it would be in the archaeologist, the rush to discover the mysteries buried for centuries to the first day And next to the signs.

Only when the psychiatrist can stick to the task of understanding, he will be free of the burden of attention to other aspects of his own professional work, such as the sympathies or antipathies provoked by certain manifestations. Neither will he fall into obfuscations similar to those incurred by another prominent professor who, without flushing, said he felt aversion to clients typified as hypochondriacs, considering them "deep egoists".

As one can well observe, moral judgments, affects and ambitions are inadvisable companies for the psychiatric exercise; but not only for the client but for the professional himself who, little by little, is distanced from the passion that, in its day, caused the beginning of the "vocation". This frustration explains the inappropriate answers and the derogatory comments of those who have in their hands the most precious thing: the person.

It is a very important question in the field of consultation, the use of language, which should be careful of which is not to be deduced from a dissimilarity between the client and the rest of the world because in short, the cabinet has to be the framework in which, in addition to finding an explanation for the ailments, the client can live an experience that repairs the damage suffered. The choice of words must be exquisitely cared for so that none can be interpreted as a new recrimination added to the already received. In this sense, one has to keep in mind that psychiatric jargon is full of nasty technicalities that reinforce the idea of exceptionality and differentiation. To show a simple example let us take the words "rehabilitation" and "reinsertion" whose use, besides being improper, refers us immediately to the Christian conception of sin, guilt and remission.

It is expected that the psychiatrist will be able to allow, without obstruction, the patient's speech, an aspect that, seeming childish -what another thing could be expected? - is not so frequent. Therefore, one of the most important conditions to be able to hold a real consultation is that the client can manifest, without restrictions, the reason that leads him there. This observation is timely in view of the frequency with which exposure may be boycotted in a variety of ways, such as emphasizing the irrational nature of complaints - a much more common method than one might think- when not appealing to moral disqualification. In short, anything that is outside the scope of the strict investigative pursuit can be considered as an artefact destined to obstruct the natural course of the story, whether or not it is a deliberate purpose.

To be in possession of inner peace is another essential factor in listening. Although it seems logical to think that this faculty should, by definition, be presumed to be present in every psychiatric practitioner, this is not so because listening is a more complicated matter than might at first, for the patient's story could easily arouses the unpleasant feeling of impotence. In addition, there is another inconvenient, no less despicable, which is that who receives it loses the leadership and this triggers not a few narcissistic resistances. Therefore, the realization of test, the diagnostic work and the eruption of the council, are frequent maneuvers designed to contain what could be an unbearable avalanche of information.

One of the sibylline procedures of containment the exposure of the sufferings is the requirement of realization of the so-called self-evaluated tests; a rude maneuver to avoid the client. Let's not say anything about certain biological tests, like the one that was in vogue years ago: the test of the suppression of dexamethasone, of which there is not even left memory. Note the gross maneuver that begins with the creation of artificial entities and then submit them to experimentation. In everyday logic it is a coarse maneuver like that of one who makes a trip to the Victoria Falls and there close his eyes and ask to the companion to describe the great show. This is what has always been happening in the psychiatric field without having to point out guilty or attribute bad intentions to anyone.

And to all this, the person, the true protagonist, is on the sidelines, when it would be so simple to allow him to speak and express his sufferings. Of course, all this, so simple and natural, would deprive the doctors of such an artificial varnish of "wise". It is thus that the psychiatrist is who has to reveal that the client is truly depressed, or not; a nonsense.

After receiving the story, the psychoanalyst uses the interpretation and its subsequent submission to the client's criteria. Because, let's not forget that the consultation is, above all, a collaboration between its two protagonists. The Interpretation is the logical consequence of the patient's story, not is a divination. Here again the common sense tells that a careful attention and the absence of pressing need for leadership, it leads to a congruent explanation.

That nature never works by jumps is accepted principle by all disciplines of knowledge. However, in the field of Psychiatry it is frequent that the client's person, even in good faith, to indicate a date or an event as the beginning of the appearance of the symptom that leads to the consultation. In relation to this it is possible to affirm that this appreciation is moved by the desire of simplification, to make things simpler, an unconscious scheme that is easily discovered in the first moments of the consultation, because behind of any manifestation there are always some remote conditioners that explain their development in the way it does. The changes which seem to burst suddenly are the consequence of a preparatory work, included the course of the infectious diseases, because every infectious process must be studied in its dialoguing character; that is, in any circumstance the effects that a pathogen agent can cause are modulated by the interaction of the two elements at issue: the infectious agent and the host with his history behind. Erroneously, it is now assumed that the result depends only on the first.

The interpretation is the tool that the psychiatrist uses to arrive at the revelation of the meaning of the symptom, which is inaccessible directly to the reasoned deduction. Interpretation, however, is not something that comes from the psychiatrist's wisdom, no; is the acquisition that, in collaboration with the client, is gradually deduced through the sessions. It is of no use, therefore, for the psychiatrist to play the role of a fortune-teller because, even if his interpretation could be correct, the benefit would be null and void and would have no other purpose than the exaltation of his vanity since it would not be endorsed by his "Insight", by his acceptance. This process of knowledge -also known as a therapeutic process- is the result of a joint effort in which all inquiry must be submitted to the rational part of the client.

The successive interpretations, if they are timely and correct -and can hardly be erroneous if they are the consequence of the patient's story-, restore the biographical contiguity broken by the action of the moral conscience during the process of education. With this, genuine personal valuation, I do not say that it would be repaired but would be established for the first time. At the same time, guilt feelings would dissipate, allowing the subsequent harmony between parties hitherto in rivalry. Because happiness, although it is an ethereal term, has a precise reality in the field of Psychology: neither more nor less than "being friends with oneself." Such is the goal to achieve, a destiny that would seem puerile at first sight but that constitutes the greatest achievement that in this life is possible to reach.

The state of enmity with oneself comes when obstacles opposing the attainment of natural aspirations convince the child that they are absurd and that those who desire such things are bad children, "different", apart from the others, "rare". And on this framework is established the true spiritual suffering, the most painful of all. To feel oneself Feeling apart from the world, exiled, is the cruelest of torments. Through the interpretation, and in the acquiescence of the client, the personal image is gradually freed from the "mistakes" conditioned by the merciless action of the past.

Those who feel an invincible anguish at the time of taking the elevator, or for whom the irruption of that unbearable sensation prevents them from undergoing the narrowness of a medical examination, such as the scanner, or those who are forced to go back over their steps, again and again, never to be totally convinced that they have left the gas key closed, to give some common examples, they will accept that there must be something explaining such "irrationality" that escapes immediate understanding. Well, that element will coincide with the unconscious content described by Freud. In its unmasking psychoanalytic work is consumed. Does it by mere whim? No, absolutely not. The person subjugated by these contents resembles the blind person located in an unknown place, without any guiding signal.

Even at the risk of appearing repetitive, I think it is necessary to insist that the interpretation should not contain any moral judgment. I insist on this because of the excessive frequency with which the misinterpretation of a behaviour results in great calamities, especially in adolescence, a time characterized by excellence of experimentation and self-assertion, frequently confused with rebellion, in which the misunderstanding of a fact can start a path without return, as in the case of experimentation with prohibited substances. Thus, what is only the satisfaction of a juvenile curiosity can become the beginning of a calvary. In this sense, it is striking how easy the elders forget their childhood and youth ages.

Another condition that seems unnecessary to emphasize is that the psychiatrist must keep the secret of everything exposed in the cabinet. Again we are facing an obvious warning, but it is that on some occasions, few by fortune, these rules are transgressed. In a process of separation, another reputed professor was unscrupulous to advise the husband's lawyer, revealing data of the professional secrecy of the wife, who had been previously his client.

After commenting on the elements present in the query we arrive at the moment of treatment, a term that I prefer to replace with the one of care, the final destination of the query. The use of the term treatment is more appropriate to describe the successive steps in the preparation of a product, such as the wine, to give an example. For this reason, I have intentionally substituted the term of treatment for that of collaboration, since psychological care, like any other company, can only be based on the agreement of parties for a cooperation in which they accept the agreed conditions. Because any plan must first be agreed upon, clearly stating the terms of the contract, the scope and limitations of it. When it is clearly established and agreed, it'll be a solid link for the collaboration of both client and doctor. On the contrary, everything that dodges in the first steps will be a hindrance that will creep along the attention.

It is not possible to establish the duration of the collaboration, although it must be long because, as has been mentioned, it is not a question of replacing the worn part of a mechanism; it's a form of rebirth in the fullest sense.

In relation to the duration of this collaboration, so criticized for ignorance of its reasons, we must be aware that the course of a process is never subjected to our needs. No matter how pressing is the need for a male successor, no king was known to try to shorten the time of gestation of the wife. Each process has its "tempo", its duration, that can't be shortened. The road that seems be longer, if chosen wisely, can lead to the goal more quickly. A greedy baker complained that his apprentices were causing a lot of trouble in the workroom, mostly due to the rush to gobble up cakes, taking advantage of the owner's carelessness. All this had the consequence that he has to dismiss them promptly and to prepare new apprentices. One night, when his daily task was over, he confided to his wife the reason for his displeasure, and she commented that "if you were not so vigilant, things would happen naturally", "What should I do, then, let them eat all the sweets?" He replied, scandalized. But she merely replied, "Do as you like" This reply bewildered the grumpy baker but he served him for to think all night long. The following day, when she received the new candidates, she said: "Before I begin the teach all of you the secrets of the trade, this week we will dedicate it entirely to eating as many sweets as you wish, in this way I will know which ones are to your liking and those that will sell better. And what had to happen, took place. The fellows filled themselves with sweets till the indigestion made hating the all sweets, ice creams, meringue and other candies. That way the baker could continue his trade in the middle of a tranquillity never before experienced.

It is possible to compare the therapeutic work with the effort of the anatomic in his patient task of releasing the different layers of tissues until exposing the structure of the organ sought or, what is the same, the fact of unravelling a ball of wool.

Moreover, the research that takes place within the framework of the therapeutic alliance is full of simplicity, as long as that the person of the psychiatrist do not be a slave of elements foreign to the task itself, such as those related to vanity. But if he can submit to the representation he has, with no other endeavors or ambitions, the task is as simple as that of those who entertain themselves by putting together the pieces of a puzzle, without asking that the world be amazed by his sagacity or his speed in the completion of the task.

From what we have said it follows that the attention must be based on an active collaboration between the two parties preceded by a covenant, just like in any other company. The approach of the conditions of collaboration is an indispensable requirement for the achievement of the desired goal. It is not one person who is going to run with responsibility of influencing the other; is the collaboration between both which will enable the discovery of the enigma hidden behind the symptom. As this collaboration progresses over the time -and here the haste is counterproductive- the dynamic forces are reorganized more effectively towards the wellbeing of the individual, always keeping in mind that before the symptom disappears there will be varied the dynamic disposition of psychic forces.

As far as the practice of psychiatry is based upon the pursuit of knowledge, it is absurd to introduce any other expression of moral connotation, such as the use of the word "help", a more appropriate term for the exercise of charity. In the collaboration of both parts, that must necessarily govern the psychoanalytic work, nobody helps to anyone. The enterprise will be carried out for the mutual benefit.

Finally, let us devote some commentary on the psychiatric formation of our universities, which worsens day by day in its everlasting struggle to be accepted in the medical sphere for what, living from the psychological -that no other thing means the psyche prefix-, incurs in the incoherence of an organicist drift. And, in accordance with this nonsense, the psychiatric units are cornered in the last plants of the general hospitals.

Such is the incongruity that dominates this panorama that, not only here but in many other universities, appear publications with the latest findings of "psychiatric research", always related to "anomalies in brain tissue", if not with "genetic alterations". And it is that informatics has come to the aid of all the lazy minds that, by transforming any data, even false, into a number, revel with statistical images, believing been, thus, truly researchers. But the thymus is easily detectable since no psychological observation can be translated into numerical data.

Research in Psychology is a fallacious exercise and the statistics applied to this field is, simply, a blunder. Because, for the preparation of statistical studies it is necessary to start from objective data, only thus it is possible to compare, to add, and to make percentages. But as far as people's lives are concerned, it is impossible to add affections and emotions and compare them, a naive maneuver done in the false belief that these operations add some kind of knowledge.

These shrewd "thinkers" use the latest achievements of computer engineering to fulfil the ambition of any every psychological "researcher": to transform observations into data, numbers and graphs. Because, besides, they start from a false premise which is the assumption that there are clearly delimited diagnostic entities, such as psychopathy, obsessional neurosis, and so on. But alas! As far as the person's manifestations are unclassifiable, this research is nothing more than an entertainment of frustrated psychologists.

Moreover, the congresses of Psychiatry are programmed in clear imitation of the medical congresses and end with the same sentence, always referred to a "last generation" drug, of which it is affirmed that "it open up unsuspected expectations" in eradication of this or that illness. In this sense, many of the academic figures who, perhaps, in the past have been of some use, roam extemporaneously the university halls, directing the anachronistic doctoral theses.

Strictly considering the facts, whatever their nature, are unrepeatable under the same conditions, even those belonging to the world of natural sciences, of physics and chemistry, in which the molecular and atomic arrangement is not the same in the repetition of successive trials; even less, with those related to the behaviours. Here, a second experiment may have similarities to the first, but it can never be exactly the same, because an experience, that was not in the past, is now included. Therefore, an investigation that does not take into account the impossibility of repeating the same test can not be considered as rigorous. At a crossroads, we will never know what would have happened if we had been free to take another road. For this reason, in spite of frequently speaking of "error", with respect to the behaviours, we ignore its sense. For in the resolution of a mathematical calculation it is possible to admit the existence of error, since the same operation can be repeated one and a thousand times under identical conditions, but never in regard to the experiences of life which take place within of an unrepeatable time frame. In consideration of this circumstance it is never advisable to accept the experiences of others as a guide to the one's own. Everyone is chained to their own adventure.

All this explains the fact that, within the confines of the psychiatrist's office, neither lie nor error makes sense, since it is impossible to know what would have happened if it could have taken another path and, even in the case of finding a plausible deduction, it could never be demonstrated. The experiences of life are unrepeatable and the choice of the path is a chimera because, at every moment, the path imposes itself.

Curiously, we speak with lightness of error, as if we were in possession of the unambiguous formula out of which everything is wrong. This, if possible, would imply two circumstances that do not exist: on the one hand, the existence of this formula and on the other, that of being in possession of the freedom to choose.

I confess to feeling displaced, alien, and strange in the world of my specialty, different from most of my colleagues, with hardly any points in common with most of them. And in this sense, this essay should be intended to sing the chasm that separates me from colleagues, "pill dispensers"; merchants of a gullible and drowsy society, better than to the disclosure of the specialty.

Fortunately, my position in the exercise of Psychology is privileged due to the knowledge of two extraordinary people: doctors Carlos González and Jerónimo Molina who opened to my eyes "Peña Retama", a miracle of clever and human attention. Imagine witnessing, from the top of a tower, how a multitude is struggling in search of an object that from the heights is clearly distinguished but that, because of the excessive proximity, they pass again and again to their side without noticing its presence. Naturally I do not boast of this circumstance which is product of the same chance that governs our lives, but the coexistence of those unrepeatable dates strengthened in me the conviction that it was what I was looking for and that the fortune, embodied in these two benefactors and their extraordinary creation, had led me there.

In every discipline, in each of the professionals who practice it and, perhaps, in the same users, however practical are their aims, as is the case of Psychology, there is an interest that transcends this same pragmatic purpose. The professional is not entirely satisfied that his activities achieve immediate results, always underlies the interest of how and through which principles are obtained, or are refused, those expectations. This is why in all studies it reserves one or more chapters that try to answer these questions. For personal satisfaction is not satisfied with the mere fact of healing or alleviation, but rather aspires to have clear awareness of the scope, limits, and the pillars that are underneath its practical activity. This is what confers security and wellness: the knowledge.

Offering gloves to those who come to the consultation for the suffering of an obsessive neurosis, which is expressed by the endless ritual of washing hands, seems a sarcasm, an absurdity for those who aspire to heal the other's ailment. Let us settle in the Middle Ages, and in the effort to put the armour to a rickety warrior without coming to the ground over his face. The most energetic preparers would repeat the operation so many times they were precise until they accustomed our victim to endure so heavy protection. Others, however, would make a parenthesis, reflect and feed conveniently this ungainly pawn, in the hope that, strengthened, he could emerge victoriously from the test. These two approaches, or different tactics, are present in a multitude of disciplines that have practical purposes; It follows that the practical is not at odds with knowledge. These two positions have important repercussions for personal fulfillment, by the satisfaction that can give a well-ordered activity. It is already known that in this business, as in any other of life, there are two opposing positions: waiting to strengthen or rush into the action without any reflection.

# 4. THE PSYCHOLOGY AND THE LIFE

Even knowing that he will not find an answer, the person will ask to himself, again and again, for the meaning of life. Psychology, which pursues an explanation of how the person is in life, would seem more compelled to find an answer, but in this search emerges the first and insurmountable obstacle. What is life? What is that flowing through the days, so full of longing hopes, passions, loves and jolts? And what is its purpose? We know nothing. And yet, no one is resigned to not having a notion about the existence. For some, it will be the opportunity to evolve, for others the test before reaching paradise, who knows! Life may be nothing more than waking up every day, just like the succession of movements of inspiration and expiration or a run after love or duty; in any case, a tempestuous arrival for a permanent farewell.

The most common is to equate life with a journey, a journey between an initial point of departure and an end point of arrival, something like an excursion, although organized by an arbitrary guide, so the characteristic feature of this trip is the uncertainty, with what most resembles an adventure full of uncertainty by the events that can occur along the route. The uncertainty is for the adventure what the pulse is for the heart. However, unlike the adventure that the explorer undertakes in search for glory through unknown places, here the trip is forced. As for the value of existence there are disparate opinions: for some, is a suggestive experience, others, however, will be of the opinion that few trips justify carrying a suitcase. So to define what life consists of is an overly ambitious task for the modest purpose of these pages.

The celebrated Mexican "corrido", "Camino de Guanajuato", starts with the taciturn stanza that reads: "Life is worthless, it always starts crying and crying it always ends". But, apart from the feeling one has of it, everyone will talk about the life as it has gone in her, as in the fair.

The impossibility of defining life, not even knowing its meaning, or the purpose pursued by the succession of the days of the people on earth, will make us contented with the commentary of its phases, universally shared, if there were not an early detention. Let us agree that Psychology deals with the study of the particular trajectory of being throughout the days of his life, of his attitude in them, his particular way of reacting to temporal events, as well as the form of their interaction with the others; because, to reduce the scope of their competence to the study of the conduction of nerve impulses or to the hypothetical genetic conditions that determine their actuation, would be a poor simplification of the rich variety of nuances of the person in her "being in the world with others".

However, it is possible to highlight some characteristics of the existence, shared by all, as well as to comment on the stages of their wandering through the days of the trip. Among the former, apart from the defencelessness, dissatisfaction occupies a pre-eminent place: the being feels constrained in subjection to its role, hence it tries to get rid of that attachment, either through evasion provided by imagination, consumption of euphoriants substances and other forms of liberation, such as those offered by the arts. Among the latter are the artificial divisions of the different moments of the evolution of being: birth, childhood, adolescence, youth, maturity, senescence, and death. All of them deserve some comments, from the psychological point of view.

Our knowledge is based on the succession of the observed phenomena, so that we come to the conclusion that each effect is preceded by a cause and this, in turn, is determined by another precursor, and so till to come to some origins that remain in the mystery. This chaining of causes and effects gives the existence its procedural character and this is how we explain the trajectory of the person throughout their existence; A route framed by the conditions, that are more determinant the closer they are to the beginnings of life and the more accessories how much closer they are to the term of the journey. This, that seems to be obvious, is ignored both in the treatises of psychiatry itself and in the essays on history due to our uncontrollable impatience to find a point from which to establish the beginning of everything; a way to gain some security.

Giving to circumstances such a decisive role in the life of the persons, it may give the impression that the leadership of these is somewhat disdained, to the point that nothing from the person himself would exert a decisive influence, nor in their individual or collective history. Should Ortega and Gasset's sentence: "I am me and my circumstances" be replaced by that of "I am only my circumstances?" This way of reasoning, which would not disgust the understanding if it were applied to the study of physical phenomena, seems insulting when used in the study of psychological facts, as Freud had already noticed with his discovering of the unconscious. The entrails of being seem to squeak before the possibility of losing a leadership that, although well thought, belongs more to the domain of faith than to reason. With this approach the vanity of being suffers a mortal blow. Because, things considered this way, the being would be mediatised by an unbearable certainty that would reduce to rubble the pillars that are holding all the civilizations, based upon the believing of the transcendence of the person. Farewell to the grandiloquent pronouncement "Alea jacta est", attributed to Julius Caesar, to whom the threat of its enemies, as much as to his own decision, determined to cross the Rubicon. Farewell, too, to the praises, honours, praises, merits and monuments.

So much depredation, should be tolerable? However, psychological analysis requires that everything that is not deductible be dispensed with, otherwise no socially unacceptable behaviour could be studied.

For all of this, it is better that in our study we separate ourselves from all transcendence with which we are accustomed to enhance the person and stick exclusively to the traits of the stages shared by all.

Probably the persons are not devoid of all faculties and, on the contrary, there is one that, not yet essentially belonging to them, does go with them throughout his career. I mean his indestructible disposition to falling in love. This inclination, which is part of the instinctive equipment with which the being accedes to life, like the defensive reflex movements, can be observed in all people, even those who embrace religious vocations and renounce worldly interests, and in each and every one of the stages of its development.

The representation of life opens in the trance of birth. It is the moment in which the new being accedes from the darkness to the light, from the comfort to the open air, from the paradise to the eviction, from the plethora to the shortage. It is not surprising, then, that the creature appears to the world, lacking the capacity for verbalization, amid sobs and erratic grimaces that we interpret as gestures of strangeness and discomfort.

It is then that our eyes open to life; a traumatic experience in which the child is pushed through a distressing channel to emerge, between whines, to a new reality. It's a forced trip without prior request or permission, because no one, as we know, was consulted before being born. Birth is an involuntary event and the beginning of an uncertain passage through a suffocating tunnel, so that in the fact of birth one might think that the person has the first experience of what we know by anguish -from the Latin language, that means narrow, narrowness-. It is not surprising, therefore, that, in the face of so much grief, the child's restlessness has been treated to appease with songs as full of tenderness as the universal lullabies, among which is specially moving the composed by the genius of Manuel de Falla.

The crying that accompanies the infant in his appearance might well be due to the fact that he had been expelled from the Eden. It is a disconsolate cry for which, in Huesca, is used a beautiful word: there it is said that the child "grama". In parentheses, despite the disruption of the child's cry, there are paediatrician colleagues who advise the parents to resist their heartbreaking cry and separate him early from the conjugal bedroom so that it becomes accustomed, in a precipitate and soulless process of growth.

With birth, nature completes its victory. But, as in every battle, there must be an adversary defeated and in this case two are defeated: on the one hand, the mother who with this act dismisses her youth and on the another, the new being who is involuntarily introduced into a medium of ungovernable bewilderment.

Like all events, birth has repercussions that affect the two planes of existence: the individual plane and that of the species; to the personal and to the social sphere. Consequently, what could interest one may disgust the other.

We find ourselves, then, with two superimposed worlds: the world of facts as they are imposed and the world of how they were wanted; two parallel interests always gravitating over the lives of people and constituting, with their confrontation, the essence of what, in his day, I gave the title "The Disease of Life".

In the same act of birth are outlined all the answers to the questions about the future personal particularities that are, in addition, the object of the Psychology,

The child who has the fortune to grow freely, under the placid and captivated look of the mother, will experience a special pleasure to walk naked, as a proud display before his lover and as a prelude to a security that will accompany him throughout his life. This authorization will mark his future and those to whom the fate has distinguished, will always walk in possession of an inexhaustible treasure. Subsequently, the obliged dresses, physical and psychological, will make these ineffable moments unrepeatable.

If the newborn had the capacity to construct some reasoning, then, once the baby has passed the trauma of birth, it would be said, "since I am here, let's see what this is about". So the forced curiosity presides over the period of childhood. Exploration is the work of the early times of the infant, an inquiry that begins with the lips, gateway to the digestive tract and that, depending on the peace that presides this moment, will leave lasting traces in its functioning. Although, more than the knowledge of the outside world, the infant is attentive to the response awakened in the mother by his awkward movements. Thus, he will continually turn his gaze to her for approval.

But it will be necessary to return on the mentioned characteristics of the birth when it is commented the lack of signification that, for the Psychology, has the term freedom.

Later, if fortune is not very adverse, this uneasiness will be appeased whenever the mother's breast approaches to his mouth: first reunion with the substitute of the lost paradise.

And here we leave the creature at the beginning of an eagerness that will never be interrupted; The indefatigable pursuit of an impossible return, which will acquire diverse appearances in successive stages, and which, as with the waves of the sea, will be an example of the struggle between the individual life and that of the species.

This brief review of the birth phase would be incomplete without mentioning the people in charge of the new being, the parents, and their particular way of being in the world. The child is pushed to a world of expectations, beginning the ordeal of education with the weaning and control of the sphincters, until its start in games in which the cleaning of clothes may be another point of application of the restrictions.

And before the desired thing, the ordeal of the schooling will begin, ideal scenario for the battle between the desire and the duty. Soon, the labels like Autism, Asperger's Syndrome and School Failure, will stick on the helpless backs of schoolchildren in a delirious competition for knowing who can be the best tamer. "Desasnar" -like to civilize the monkey- was the term used to describe the task that was presented to the teachers before the arrival of new students.

The calamitous state of education is a consequence, among other factors, of the confusion between the boundaries of teaching and education. To the first belongs the transmission of data, delimited and objective, and generally subject to political changes; to education, discipline much more ambitious than the first, all the baggage that the person receives because of being a social creature and that has in the family frame the initial and determining classroom. In teaching is the repetitive effort of data by which the student stores it is in his memory. Teaching involves an active and constant attitude, in line with the abilities of the students and throughout the duration of the class.

This, which seems obvious, is in practice disregarded. This is the only way to understand that from childhood the child is transported a saddlebag full of books in a constant come and go, no matter what, in the middle of an absurd school schedule -often longer than the working hours- that keeps confined In the desk the creatures irresistibly attracted by the game and the physical activity.

Extemporaneous is also the delay in the incorporation of electronic means that would lighten the heavy backpacks that mistreat their vertebral columns. It is extraordinary the teaching's ability to transform the pleasant in annoying. And, to top it all, the study plans, which could have permanently preserved the numbering of the different courses like first, second, etc., have undergone as many changes as the ministries of education. Thus we have the EGB. ESO, etc.

It is difficult to understand the extraordinary and noisy controversy around the subject of education, only explicable by seeing in it an environment conducive to the satisfaction of editorial interests, political indoctrination and passivity of teachers, who spend hours in endless speculation. All these factors can turn teaching simplicity into an impossible undertaking. New plans follow each other, year by year, depending on the governments on duty.

If one look at the fact that, finally, what remains from the secondary school are just four data, we would recognize that teaching can be a company easily accessible. On the other hand, presenting it full of complexity has the purpose of justifying the repeated failure of countless plans of study. And, in the end, it will ultimately be decreed that the student is to blame for the unfortunate state of this affairs.

Focusing on the theme with dispassion, we will agree that subjection to school discipline is mortification for any child. Whoever believes otherwise has only to wait for the passage of time because, as long as the child has strength, he will do everything possible to please the wishes of his parents, but this does not mean that there is only one child who wants to go to the school, so that, with this factor in mind, and taking into account that the school period is part of the many difficulties that life presents, it should be established that the substantial part of this difficulty must be borne by teachers. They are the ones who must capture the particular situation of each student and, according to that, develop the teaching activity. Does the child learn to talk by going to a class? No, the incessant repetition of the words coming out of the mother's mouth is doing the work. Therefore, the strenuous activity of repetition, together with the purpose of not leaving behind any student, should constitute the soul of teaching.

But, oblivious to this effort, the teachers wander through the institutes, wasting time in sterile meetings, when not in tutoring or in subpoenas to parents who, besides pleasing the vanity of the teaching staff, alter the familiar coexistence and add new reasons of concern, in a protagonism that, in short, has nothing to do with the eagerness of teaching which, in itself, consists of nothing but indefatigable repetitions. Teaching is a matter of repetition as any other acquisition of knowledge. Certainly this endeavor requires a certain discipline but this must begin with the teacher, never with the student. In my opinion, the attitudes of teachers, their tendency to speculation, their inclination to impose their own ideas, their passivity, in fine, explain the evils that afflict the teaching. Wherever the example does not come, words are like water poured on a mat.

And if all these follies were not enough, the homework, that sly way to avoid the laborious duty, disturbing the family coexistence, complete the mess of teaching. The insistent repetition is the utensil of teaching, indispensable for all the acquisitions called to leave a substrate in the memory. It is through the diligent repetition of the mother as the child acquires the capacity of language. The home works are Machiavellian maneuvers aimed at mastery of the family by the teachers and the nesting of bitter disagreements.

Another factor which hinders the process of teaching is the excessive role of the teacher who believes that the mere repetition of data diminishes their merits, in the idea that the mere subjection to the role entrusted confines him to anonymity. But reality is which is and is not another. We all "acquire" a commitment to society by accepting a role and this has to set limits to the habitual tendency to the narcissism that, in the field of education, is particularly exorbitant.

Something similar happens to the historians, who feeling irrelevant with the mere accumulation of data, jumps over the pulpit of interpretation. Moreover, the teachers should find an intimate satisfaction in being an author of the transmission of the knowledge proposed by the teaching plans. And if any frustration was left behind, they should compensate it in their private life. Only in this way would they cease to waste hours and efforts in useless meetings and inquiries about the inscrutable sex of the angels.

The plane pilot never comes to ask the passengers how to make the landing maneuver, which is a natural thing. Why, then, are we not surprised to be required to assist teachers in the performance of their function? For, this is the message that the families receive from those who are in the charge of teaching our children. For that trip, few saddlebags are necessary. Moreover, the family, like poor dependents, is asked to attend meetings without respect to their own needs. It is another form of tyranny that is hidden under the fear of any possible revenge.

Being all of this so serious, it is still more the insolence of many educators who, breaking the limits of their representation, invade irresponsibly the field of a misunderstood Psychology to assess behaviours. Due to it, the damage that the family receives is tremendous. The so-called School Failure is none other than teacher failure. For, if we think about it, failure does not exist in the people's lives. There will be a mismatch with expectations, a greater or lesser success in calculating the forces for the achievement of forecasts, but never a failure. Let's think well about it before we speak of failure, because at the time we do it we are insulting the child and that is, in itself, a tremendous iniquity.

We could do an experiment: to select the most "outstanding" students from different schools and make a new group with them. Soon, we would find the same result: someone would occupy the top of the class and someone else the last. Unfortunately some similar experiment has been put into practice with so-called "gifted" groups, with catastrophic results, I suppose. It is embarrassing to think that in a recent past centers have been created for these children, and even more shameful is that no voice had risen before such an aberration.

And it is that every human group is susceptible of being classified, from first to last, according to these mistaken assumptions. But does this mean that we should discard from society those who occupied the last places? In addition, life is a vast area of interests and the academic success occupies only one place among many others.

The punishment agrees to the education as much as the nakedness to the cold winter. The learning process follows the same steps as the rest of the activities in which there is an initial difficulty to overcome but which, once overcome with kindness, becomes an engine that drags until completing the acquisition of the material to be incorporated. Something similar to what happens in the reading of novels that its first pages would lack of any attraction but that, as the development of the plot goes on, the curiosity subjugates the reader until the end of the book.

From time to time the Psychology goes out of its boundaries and collaborates with the teaching for perverse ends, such is the case of the called Asperger Syndrome, picture characterized by the curious sympathy that the student experiences towards a certain subject and to the detriment of the rest that abandons irremissibly. Well, Psychology has found in this behaviour a new find to which to put a title: Asperger Syndrome. I wonder: but, have we all felt the same attraction towards all the subjects of the school year or, on the contrary, have we felt an open antipathy for one of them? Undoubtedly this behaviour cannot be understood under this ingenuity but as the expression of a more complex question.

There are authors, such as Ricardo Moreno, who, in my opinion very aptly, attributes to the proliferation of new specialties, such as pedagogy, the germ of evil that undergoes the teaching. Sarcastically he speaks of this profession as the absurdity of learning to "teach to teach." Of course the same could be said of the "political scientist", the "environmentalist" and other modern "specialties" that so generously lavishes the science of our days.

Social pressure, on the other hand, makes the parents feel obliged to push their children towards brilliant qualifications as a guarantee of their future success -and their own tranquillity-, if not for the satisfaction of their own vanity. But since the interests of life are broad, we will understand that, at best, this success would always be partial and generally ephemeral. In any case, nothing would have to do with the purposes of Psychology that deals with the harmonious development of all faculties of the individual in order to achieve their maximum level of well-being. About this observation, it seems appropriate to remember the wise gypsy saying: "I do not want to see my children with good principles". In children, as in cereals, the anticipation of the summer heat ruins the harvest. Life shows us frequent examples of dazzling beginnings but that, when adolescence arrives, they experience a dramatic detention, an exhaustion of the desire to live.

Is it timely to create a "science" to be able to understand what is directly and universally available to the observation? Does it make sense that any person be named a "specialist" in matters of all known? Psychology has no need of technicalities to make itself understood and when it does, as in the case of the coining of the ugly name "resilience" -term proposed to refer to personal ability to overcome a circumstance especially high-pitched-, not has succeeded doing the things less complicated. Therefore, better than the Lord help us when we stumbled across these sages of new stamp who dare to ensure that children will be violent if not are taught to accept a NO and that in cases of aggression from children to parents the explanation is that of a gentle education. And all this is due to the fact that education is the application of a set of tools for the observation and correction, to achieve a predetermined goal. But, the set of healthy performances are not learned in any manual but flow spontaneously to the fire of the acceptance and affection.

We leave the school stage and continue with the one that, inadvertently, has been releasing away from the young. Is the adolescence, with spectacular body modification and the emergence of new and the overwhelming impulses. At this moment the phenomenon of the "falling in love" captures all the interests of the young people. After of an imperceptible mental unrest, a persistent and diffuse fantasy crystallizes in the appearance of the "first love", which surprises the young man by subjugating his thoughts around the dreams in which a central figure occupies his enchantment.

And takes place something similar to that happens in the shooting of certain films in which the director removes the light from the general plane to concentrate it in a partial scene that, thus, is emphasized and isolated of the rest. This same isolation is the one that encapsulates the lovers who, like little dormouses, hibernate feeding their dreams, abstracted from the surrounding world.

Such a prodigy, that we usually place in the adolescence, accompanies the person throughout his existence, from birth to death, although under various appearances and manifestations.

It is a moment full of magic because the destiny of so much rapture does not exist in the reality, but is the mere prolongation of the dreamer's uncontrollable hopes. There is no other occasion in life in which the will of the person is so triumphant and that the desire and achievement coincide, although on most occasions there is no real knowledge of the beloved. This fact anticipates the consideration of that love and knowledge do not necessarily have to walk hand in hand, because in the minds of lovers is already all the characteristics that is supposed exist in the nebulous object of love.

After the first dealings with the object of love, the conflicts arise and the lovers see vanish the dream of the fusion of both in one person. Discovered the veil, the routine of life causes the inevitable encounter with what we usually call reality that, in turn, explains that the snub is the frequent end of first love.

At the end of the journey, the luckiest will be the ones who can exclaim, even to themselves: "My friend, hand in hand we have faced the gales and traps of the road. So thus it has become more bearable. And that's why I love you".

The subsequent relations will lack the splendour of the first, but they will act upon our dreamy quixotic in the same way as the bacteria in its successive passages through the guinea pigs: stripping them of much of their virulence and adjusting them better to the needs. It is the triumph of nature over the individual who has been allowed to play, for a short time, before to claim him to the fold, for to attend the mandate of conservation of the species. However, in the shadow, sneaking, like a goblin, will forever remain the charm from dawn to first love.

It seems to be a game, and certainly it may be, the parenthesis of an illusion through which the individual can satisfy the vanity of believing himself protagonist, since it is certainly only a piece of the gigantic puzzle of life. It may be a trap because the first love is not that which the lover attributes to it, but the updating of another that took place well before adolescence; may be the regrowth of the another one who remains drowsy in the confines of the heart and that could well be a sham of the love for the first person that appears in the sight of the new being: the mother.

Although the process of individuation begins with life itself, it is at this stage when the powerful centrifugal forces manifest themselves vigorously. It seems as if nature repeated the words of the gospel: "Thou shall leave thy house, and follow me". At this stage are awaken the natural forces of rebellion, indispensable in all the movements towards individuation, are also evident and, in situations in which this activity is seriously hampered, is manifested by acts of great violence which, in turn, constitute the habitual Indications for psychiatric examinations.

When one of these overwhelming events occurs, as in the parricides, there is a social confusion in the absence of an explanation of facts that appear to contradict nature itself. In this confusion, the judge calls in his aid to the psychiatrist who, in turn, is forced to jump the boundaries of his competence for support the opinion about the guilt or innocence of the author.

Basically, adolescence is an impatient waiting for the advent of adulthood, which promises independence and happiness. At this point, the fate of the person is similar to that of the donkey who walks after an unattainable carrot and that being near to achieve his purpose, another one is proposed to it. In any case, the magic of falling in love, the dream that will occupy the rest of life, is reactivated with unusual impetus at this stage. Thus, the newly arrived gallant will become the intrepid blue prince and the incipient damsel will wait for the kiss to wake her from her long dream. In the pursuit of this longing, crystallized in the achievement of a partner with whom to pass the life, they will leave the home, in the conviction that there is a soul mate waiting for the liberating kiss.

In addition, falling in love, as has been said, is universally present in all creatures regardless of social status, age, or role to represent. It may be that its manifestation, by the effect of repressive forces, is not ostensible, as is the case of religious professions, in which the object of love is displaced towards some religious figure. It is discussed if this maneuver, which is unconscious and that in Psychology receives the name of sublimation, accomplishes the pursued end. Useless discussion: the achievements in the life are volatile and all are fulfilled with the simple fact of accompanying us in the days of life. Frequent abuses in boarding schools speak of the fact that sublimation does not wipe out the violence of the instinct drive. The superb literary production of Spanish mysticism, on the contrary, shows that the drives found a more appropriate arrangement. In any case, the commitment of nature, the true purpose of falling in love, is snubbed. But, life leaves thus so many longings..!

In his essay "Love, Women and Death," Schopenhauer expresses the idea that falling in love is the disguise under which the will of nature is hidden by its permanence and, thus, describes to the pair of lovers as evildoers, conspiring in favor of the plans of procreation. Starting from this thesis, the author pleads for the annulment of the "will to live", origin of human suffering although, as we will see later, the capacity of being to opt is a mere mirage.

Aside from the fact that the falling in love, may serves as a concealment for the purposes of nature, it could be, on a deeper plane, a vehicle for something even more sublime, sadder, or more lyrical, if one wants: for the imperishable longings to return to the bosom of the mother. The frequency with which lovers express their displeasure because the couple has previously had another love, the need to be unique, apart from its undeniable usefulness to the care of the offspring, is another argument in favor of return. Famous storytellers, such as Peter Pan, testify to the probable existence of the yearning for the return to yesterday and the disgust for being swept away by the whirlwind of life.

The first love can remain or to experiment changes in relation to the object, but whatever its course will have as its purpose the formation of the couple.

If delicate is the work of the mother with the children, which is to do as the stream that is generously poured into another tributary, impossible is to make of two people one, as is the initial pretension of lovers. Is for this reason that after the initial fever has passed, the inevitable manifestations of disenchantment begin. It may be that to this disappointment refers the complaint contained in Machado's verses, "I loved as much as they can have of hospitable", equally applicable to both components of the couple.

Again here we can observe the true role of the person, who is none other than that of subordination to the superior purposes of the species. The same loving game, that begins with the usual protests of whether "you love me or not", contains the seed of disillusionment.

The uncontrollable thrust of nature causes that the repeated word "to love" has past smuggled the benevolent frontier that cross the commodities referred to the Issues of love, regardless of its precise psychological sense, cleared by Freud. This author differentiates two types of relationship: the narcissistic one, in which the person is unable to separate his needs of the source from which expects the satisfaction and another, also called "of the object", which takes into account the existence of the other, as an separate object, with its own needs and expectations. Typical example of the first is the baby who still can not to distinguish between him and the mother's breast. On the contrary, wanting, in the evolved sense of the term, implies the ability to feel some kind of affection towards someone, with the clear awareness that is different and knowing that should be no purpose of dominion or modification.

That is why the couple, or walks towards the establishment of bonds of friendship as two loyal partners in the enterprise of the care of the children or will go right towards its dissolution, because its course, of not opting for friendship, will be poisoned by quarrels, reproaches and hatreds.

Once the infatuation has fulfilled its mission, the whirlwind of daily life will drag the characters. Reluctantly, they will attend to the payment of the mortgage, the bills of light and other trivialities, until that the miracle of the birth of their children adjusts them in the assigned role.

Being in these, maturity arrives, which coincides with the work stage and here time slips insensibly, as in a sigh, until retirement. The attention to occupy a position that satisfies, at the same time, the family needs and the part of surplus vanity, will capture all the interest. Past and future are equidistant at this stage. The days slip fast in the belief of being immersed in a transcendental task, when the reality is that everything is already done. The great dreams and great fears lose, also, the impetuosity of the days gone by.

The maturity, unfortunate expression, more suitable to qualify the fruit, dismisses the youth and delves into the age of spare parts (glasses, teeth, etc.) in which we says farewell to parts that have been our partners. And, before saying goodbye, it seems sensible to think that the person should be used to these tasks; but it is not so, perhaps because the idea of the end surpasses the limits of our understanding.

For Psychology, the development of the person is already completed at this stage and few manifestations, including the ways to react to traumatic events, can be understood without taking into account the facts of the past for, due to the procedural nature of life, no one becomes different from what he was after an event however shocking it was. It is erroneously commented that Empress Sissi suffered a severe picture of anorexia-bulimia due to the rigidity of the court protocol. According to this naive conjecture, the palace should be full of feeding's alterations.

Of the same tools that the archaeologist uses to access times lost in time, makes use the psychologist to go where memory can't get. I am referring to the deduction based on indirect evidence. In every asylum one can contemplate daily the same touching spectacle of some old people who will have forgotten if they took food that same day, if they ever married and had children, if it is spring or summer, if it is day or night, but that will inevitably ask, expectantly, if his mother has already returned from her purchase. The mother is the perennial female parked in the corner of longings for the requirements of existence, but never forgotten. It may well be that the sense of the lucky bullfighting expression of "querencia" could serve to understand the way in which the old man sought shelter in the early scenes of his life. In the same way, at the end of existence, the old people direct their gaze looking for the mother. They say that Hitler, the character who frightened the world, was found dead with the photograph of the mother in his hands. I do not know how much truth is in it but is more than credible because this sublime personage, first, and perhaps unique, opportunity to have an unconditional ally, has a perennial resonance.

If not all, many of the diagnostics, object of psychiatric care, such as anorexia, bulimia and drug addiction, make immediate appeal to these anxieties of returning to the mother. The being is born from the mother, walks along looking for someone who seems to be a good substitute of her, until that, finally, returns to her in the arms of death. The longing of the returning is omnipresent.

It is by this consideration that, if it were possible to have some capacity to obtain teaching of the experience, the assimilation of separation would constitute the supreme learning of the career of life.

The fact is that one day will come the time of goodbye and behind will have remained anxieties and dreams. In that inclination that we humans have to simplify in a quality the complexity of a set, I have had for me that life is a perpetual farewell, since already from the cradle we are intoning the goodbye. Childhood takes leave of the arms of the mother, the youth of the childhood and so on, moved by the eagerness to reach a goal that, then, is revealed nonexistent, a mirage. People should be an expert in farewells; Yes, but the truth is that they are events to what no one gets used to it.

This commentary, which may seem somewhat gloomy, is compatible with the fact that in life one can also experience moments of joy, mainly due to the contemplation of the arts and the beauty of nature, which always impresses us by its greatness, in striking contrast to our insignificance.

It is not my intention to show a sombre face of existence. Optimism and pessimism are two psychologically words empty of content, which only acquire meaning in relation to expectations and desires, temptations to which no one can escape. For if we were truly free, the spiritual suffering we can observe in obsessions, delusions, and hallucinations would be meaningless. Neither should the sufferings due to separations and disappointments, because we could include these events among the natural facts of existence, beyond our control.

As the leaves of the calendar fall, so too cautiously, it begins the sliding by the slope that leads to the sunset. Gradually, steadfastness gives way to hesitancy and the interest to the indifference. The actor becomes a spectator and thus, enters the region of decline, in senescence. Just as in childhood the days seem endless, at this age they are elusive, like fish fresh out of the water.

This period of life is euphemistically known as the third age, as it is done with many other uncomfortable situations, such as the disability that is preferred to call disability, always clarifying that disability is not synonymous with less validity -it causes terror to call things by their true name, as if we had some participation in their existence-. It is the phase in which the physical capacities experience a gradual decrease, as it does the interest in the events of everyday life which up to here have occupied the forefront of attention. A particular state, a mixture of strangeness and indifference, invades the mood. It stops participating and in the eyes of this bewildered spectator the behaviours seem absurd. And is due for the train is approaching to its final station.

If fortune has allowed you to live the successive years in harmony with its requirements, you will not sink in despair the passage of the days because by then you will be vaccinated; You will know life and you will know what it can give of itself. On the contrary, that life steals you the experiences of its different stages, apart from the pertinent frustration, will incorporate in you the terrible doubt of not being clever enough, being clumsy, different from others, which is the supreme damage that a being can suffer.

In these years life is experienced as the navigator contemplates the shore to which he never will return. Memories, loves, nostalgias, hatreds and passions in general, have been weakened and the person is no longer concerned with the interests with the same urgency that he did yesterday.

When young, we see death as an event reserved for others despite the, almost clandestine, disappearance of close people. Nothing apart from the basis of the first moments of life can help us as a preparation for a serene acceptance of death as the final station of the journey.

An indeterminate date marks the turning point in the graph of life and as in the roller coaster when we culminate that disturbing rise, what remains is the dizzying descent up to the detention. The equidistance between the magnitudes of yesterday and tomorrow disappears in favor of the past. Surreptitiously, the idea of the end, which accompanies the person up to his final goodbye, is into the mind to the point that it can be said that the days of senescence are spent shepherding the dead, while the physical faculties decline, the freshness of the skin is withered, the gray hair invades the scarce mass and the pieces are replaced by other artificial ones. The prosthetic age has arrived. The sticks hold what, until recently, the limbs ruled arrogantly, the glasses try to alleviate the diminution of visual acuity, the sound amplifiers try to hold us to the environment, while the interest, like a stream, is precipitated into the sea of the childhood's days.

The fact is that one day comes the moment of final goodbye.

And death, which has always been considered as the natural outcome of life, has been reduced, in these times, to a mere disease that science has been unable to avoid, a medical failure. It is a sort of arrogance, that has its impact, in addition, in the doctor's offices in which the doctor-patient dynamics has undergone a modification of one hundred and eighty degrees; Submissive and respectful only a few days ago, full of arrogance today. All diseases have to get a healing, so that the death must to be, simply, a failure of medicine.

Of nothing has been worth the experience of having attended to the funerals of some near beings, nor the experience of have been shivering before the repeated "Dies Irae." No, life can't end of this so silly way, nor any other way. How is it possible that once reached the moon we can't ford this difficulty? How is it possible today, that we change hearts, livers, kidneys and we produce drugs against the aging?

But life does not belong to us; it is an illusory property that any mishap can snatch. For whom the conditions of the life have forced to the deviation of "his way" or to postpone the realization of the desires within his reach, he will experience death as the plunder that Seneca refers to.

With this senseless pride installed in the minds, the multiple references to death, such as the song that Carmen Linares sings: "The one that is considered himself as a great, that goes to the cemetery and there will see what the world is, in a span of land", are of little value.

Those whose days of existence hadn't permit to storage any patrimony, either in the form of a hobby or any kind of playful inclination, do not expect to start, in the final stage of life, activities that the urgencies of the existence had forced to postpone, because the deadlines for its start have already expired. It is often to hear comments of people that expect, at the time of his retirement, to begin the cultivation of tastes that could not have been attended, but it is as much the as demanding a provision for which there has not been the corresponding payment.

The life is comparable to any economic system. In relation to affections and feelings, no one can invent any that does not form part of their biographical patrimony, no matter how much advise it the moral and social conventions; where there is nothing, nothing can be drawn, although these affects even related to the parents. The affection flows joyously towards the people with whom the coexistence has been presided over by the signs of the friendship; on the contrary, from those who one has suffered outrages, one may, at most, verbally express an affection while in the heart will nest the resentment. To force oneself to love those who hate oneself is the most effective way to rush into ruin. Again here we find the proof of the dissociation that can exist between the moral and individual planes.

When a significant being leaves us, the natural reaction is the grief, the sadness, the blackness of thought. The farewell of loved ones will be as complex as complicated have been the relationships along the days of life. If they were turbulent, agitated will be likewise the farewell; if pleasant, restful will be the goodbye. In the first case, the accounts were maladjusted, ordered in the second.

But, when moral considerations forces to feel an affection that the passage of days has not left in the heart, It happens what it is known, in Psychiatry, with the inadequate diagnosis of "pathological grief", which refers to the persistent adherence to farewells that never ends. Given that the conditions of life are those that establish these modalities of farewells, it is grotesque to describe as pathological these behaviours, on the other hand as frequent, as those people who flock day after day to the tomb of the "beloved ones", in a striking scene which, contemplated as a spectator, can be attributed more to subjugation than to affection.

For this reason, to speak of pathological mourning can only obey to the fatuity of baptizing a fact with a technical name which, on the other hand, is not more than the result of an impeded development. Similarly as, years ago, it was titled with the lamentable name of "vigorexia" to the incoercible passion for bodybuilding.

Bearing in mind that it is necessity that drives every human movement, it will be a natural consequence that the yearning to be free of it is the engine of all striving. The cultivation of philosophy neither escapes from the longing to find, in the wisdom, the way to make more bearable the helplessness that governs this valley of tears.

Without losing sight of the aforementioned procedural nature of life and the involuntary nature of our arrival into the world, we will easily understand that the much-vaunted freedom, of which we have sometimes boasted, is nothing more than an illusion. In spite of our pride, we are nothing different from the insignificant autumnal leaf that, detached from the tree and blown by the wind, is precipitated in the whimsical currents of the stream.

The life of people depends on two forces: one that pushes forward and another that sucks from the end. As a medical student, we followed the text of a celebrated author, Morros Sardá who, in order to explain the movement of blood through the circulatory stream, used the simple scheme of the combined action of two complementary forces: an impelling one, due to ventricular contraction, called "vis-a-tergo", and another one, aspirant, known as vis-a-fronte, sucking it back into the atria. Freud would follow this same scheme by referring to the instinctive forces that accompany the individual throughout the days of life. At first, the motor of life, he would call Eros, which would correspond with the "vis-a-tergo", and at the second, the sucker would call it Thanatos, which would correspond with the "vis-a-fronte"; two instincts present in the adventure of existence: Eros and Thanatos. If we were to customize the driving force we would do it in the figure of the mother, the safe port where the child arrives, sleepwalking and terrified, when pressed by nightmares; if we were to represent the instinct of Thanatos, we would also do it in the mother, in the more or less concealed aspiration to return to her. In the mother come together the life and the secret yearning for to returning to her, to the eternal, to nothingness.

If the person had any capacity to vary his life trajectory, we could distinguish two classes of adventurers: some who hope to arrive safely at a predetermined destination and others open to everything that the adventure will offer to them. This last provision is established only with the passage of the years or after the overcoming of serious cataclysms, reason why the possession of a stoic aptitude does not depend on our will since, among other things, the term will is simply a psychologically hollow term. People's lives follow the same path as bodies in a vacuum: the initial impulse will determine its movement, and its persistence will last until an opposing force stops it. We can speak of fatality or fate, but hardly of will or capacity of management. Rationally considered, the life of the people is not a story of good and bad people, except that this only has the purpose of a provisional relief. Civilization, the evolution of man, is the struggle for the unattainable conquest of homeostasis, for the achievement of absence of tension, and in this purpose we are all passive subjects in the performance of the role assigned by life.

# 5. RELATED TOPICS

As has already been said, the present presentation on psychiatric discipline has nothing to do with the controversies aroused by the attractiveness of this subject. These lines do not defend or stand against any orientation of the many that in this field coexist, but are the particular exposition of my opinions stored in the prolonged exercise of this discipline. It is like a feeling, comparable to the product of any distillation whose content can be condensed in the following way: the commitment in the greatest possible approximation to the understanding of how the person in the world is. Secondarily is the source of the greatest satisfaction in the exercise of the profession. In no way pursues the elaboration of a catalogue of advice, norms or tactics that would make the existence of the client's trajectory more bearable. In this sense, the course of the days has moved me from an interventionist position to another expectant and researcher, once proven the futility of the first.

In my opinion, the appeal to ethical, moral, religious rules and, in general, the use of qualifications and recommendations, denaturalizes the psychological procedure. The exclusive principle that should govern psychological activity is to pursue a coherent explanation for both, psychologist and client, the conditions that explain the particular position of the person in the world and inseparably to this task will also be interested in offering my own opinion of their own about the main conditions that accompany him throughout the life.

### 5.1. Sex

It is the engine that has moved humanity from the caves to the present day and presumably will continue doing it, although in the present day it is importance seems to be discovering. Without the need for any special knowledge, with the sole observation, it follows that they are designed to carry out the reproductive function. Moreover, the irrepressible sexual instinct, the Eros, will make unnecessary academic preparation for the enjoyment of the fun associated with the propagation of the species, although at the present time it is preached the convenience of following a manual or putting oneself in hands of an "expert".

Every event in life, no matter how insignificant it may seem, has its repercussion, such is said to be the case of the flapping of a butterfly that moves the entire universe, even if it is in infinitesimal values. In this sense, the works of Masters and Johnson I have always considered banal to me because they add nothing to knowledge in itself. However, in the weakening of the taboo that has meant everything concerning with sex, has been of great importance. Because it cannot be denied that education has been a powerful brake on the expression of the sexual through the formation of the moral conscience, to the superego. But what is said, the need to "learn" or "teach" the mechanics of procreation is as useless pursuit as training the eyelids in their protective work of the opening and closing movement of the eyeballs. What is instinctive does not require any learning.

A different thing is that the evolution of mankind has made it necessary to put a bridle on the most powerful instincts, perhaps to channel the powerful energies in the attainment of the ends of survival. Something similar to the function of the dam that restrains the impetus of the river in benefit of other profits. But this restraint can't be interpreted as the whim of a perverse mind that handles the threads of human existence, like so often one tends to trivialize. The meaning of the plans of life surpasses the human understanding.

Psychiatry, unlike anatomy and physiology, is only exceptionally called for the writing of arrogant opinions about sexual function.

On the other hand, we remember that until very recently homosexuality was considered as a disease, in what is rare and anomalous that has the term disease. To enter into the discussion of whether the couple composed of persons of the same sex are marriage, or not, is something alien to the psychological understanding since the term marriage has its definition and this ditch all discussion, reason why the irruption on this contest of some representative of psychiatric discipline is a sheer nonsense. Rely on the respect that infuses this specialty to impose judgments unrelated to the task of the specialty is, simply, an intellectual outrage.

But the subject of homosexuality and, above all, the interest in qualifying as a marriage the union of two persons of the same sex is clear that it obeys to other aspirations other than those of knowledge. Not so the subject of the improperly called "free choice of sexual orientation," which is of enormous scientific and philosophical interest, since again here beats the controversial issue of freedom.

Psychiatric discipline has nothing to do with the recent movements and controversies raised by the issue of "voluntary choice of sexual orientation". Let us not forget that the purpose of this treatise is the disclosure of the principle that governs it, which is none other than that of the understanding. When, as in this field, morality, justice, historical remnants and other considerations that make this subject are mixed, we must confine ourselves to saying that, following the anatomical knowledge, the morphology of the sexual organs seems to have been "conceived" with reproductive purposes. It happens, however, that since this function is inseparably associated with the enjoyment of the greatest pleasure, sexuality can be a source for the satisfaction of many other interests, such as legitimate social claims, the confrontation of the sexes, and so on.

To the Psychology belongs, only, to the study of the person in the reality that he has, not in what he believes he should have. Everything else, such as pride in the voluntary choice of a particular sexual role, should be understood as being part of any other type of behaviour, knowing that no one chooses the sexual pattern, neither being high or low, sympathetic or unpleasant. In the purported choice of sexual role, there is no room for pride or repentance. The sexual role, like any other personal position, is determined by the circumstances present in the process of education and development.

The fact that homosexuality has recently been excluded from the catalogue of mental illness does not mean that Psychology, understood as a discipline in charge of understanding human behaviour, disengages from the study of the sufferings of the person in which exists this particularity, as neither it would disdain the study of a person by having blonde hair: simply, will be limited to receive any person who wants to know their evolution, without cuts, until explaining their particular way of being in life.

In any case, psychology can never chant the declarations intended to judge the sexuality, such as those that took place in recent and unfortunate manifestations of a high dignitary of the religious hierarchy, in which he affirmed that "homosexuality is a deficient sexuality", adding, not content with it, the barbarity that "pointing out a deficiency is not an offense but an aid because many cases of homosexuality can be recovered and normalized with appropriate treatment". These manifestations clearly evidence the idea they have about sexuality, normality, treatment and recovery. With regard to the treatment, I have already stated my opinion; about the recovery I invite the reader, if anyone, to ask to himself: if it has been established that life is a process, like a chain without a solution of continuity ¿how, then, is it possible to find any sense to the term recovery?

Let us recover the common sense and understand that the form in which the sexuality is manifested, it is not by a punctual choice but the culmination of the delicate process of development of the individual. Only in the case that involuntary sexual orientation was cause for suffering, and just at the request of the person, would the psychologist be allowed to exercise his profession.

## 5.2. Freedom and Will

In any matter of knowledge, the existence, or not, of what we mean by freedom is, in itself, a matter of the greatest transcendence. In the world of psychology, starting from the principle of causality in which facts are linked to other precedents, in a chain that begins at birth and in which event the child is a mere spectator, it can be anticipated that the freedom is just a mere illusion. Since every act starts from an initial impulse -which, in psychology we know by the name of motivation- a set of hidden motives to consciousness, which impels a certain action- the existence of freedom is at least questionable. Motivation is involuntary even though the person is dominated by the need to believe that he decides, although in reality he never does, because life is comparable to the trip, by train. Of a child who has received the ticket and who to the most than he can aspire is to receive the impressions of the landscape and to observe what happens in the wagon; but the destiny is just already settled beforehand and the margins of its movements are circumscribed to the limits of the compartment itself.

Can the waters choose the place where the river joins the sea? Is it allowed to the leaf, back in the autumn, to choose the place where to rest? Do the birds decide the direction of their emigration? Does the child choose the belly where to wait for the dawn of its existence? On what basis, then, does the belief that man could determine or modify the route of his journey?

The existence of some mental states, such as the obsessive and compulsive, consequent of the struggle between unconscious forces, speaks in favor of the absence of freedom and, of course, discard the assertion that the person is governed by the intelligence and the judgment. Otherwise, the reason would avoid the suffering of such bitter torments.

The existence of free will, the power to freely choose, without restriction, presupposes as much as to attain the divinity, as to be born without necessity, to be self-sufficient. Thus, any movement would be outside the law of causality for which everything has a producing antecedent and is, in turn, precursor of an effect. The denial of such a faculty means that everything is determined by the conditioning factors that make up the personal equipment along the biographical path.

On what basis, then, could the usual moral references such as praise, merit, responsibility, vice, and virtue be supported?

That the person should be free because freedom is a necessary condition for moral conscience, is an argumentation as fragile like the justification of the existence of another life, beyond this one, over the person's hypothetical yearning for transcendence. In addition, there is as much variety of moral consciences as individuals, since these are the final result, the sediment, of the educational process. If things were so artificially established, the moral conscience should contain the freedom, the possibility of follow to moral rules by all and always. But the reality shows that this is not fulfilled.

Therefore, if freedom is an illusion, as well it will be the belief of the person in a protagonism outside of being a mere actor of the role assigned by the life, so that the assumption that human endeavours, rather than being consequences of personal decisions, are nothing more than impositions of the destiny. Hence that responsibility and guilt are intellectual extravagances.

In pursuit of the laws that govern any process there is no room for the existence of freedom since otherwise it would happen that nothing could be foreseen and any experimentation could conclude with unexpected results. For Psychology, as for any other branch of science, the existence of freedom is itself a categorical impossibility.

Taking into account the models of Mechanics, we

can establish a parallelism between the laws governing the movement of bodies and the lives of people. Both begin their journey driven by an initial force, variable in both cases, and without any ability to alter either their trajectory or their speed, which is determined by the impulsion principles. The friction and the gravitation, responsible for that the movement of the objects is not perpetual we can equate them to the action of the environmental factors.

By itself, a body can't change its trajectory unless it receives the effect of an external force. Why, then, do we think that the person could voluntarily change his or her life trajectory? It would be objected that one can not equate the person with a simple physical body, which has enough springs to change its trajectory. You can even put the simple example of choosing a movie when it comes to going to the movies. But how do you evaluate the motives that lead to a particular decision? In the same way that freedom is defended at the time of the election can be questioned why some alternative has been discarded. How to assert that tastes do not play an important role in the decision? And is it possible to consider the acquisition of the tastes and hobbies regardless of the vital trajectory?

All psychological study has to start from the premise that the concept of freedom belongs to another different matter, such as religion, morality or politics. In this respect, it is classic the saying that Copernicus, Darwin and Freud humiliated the pride of mankind since, after their observations, their habitat, the earth, ceased to occupy the center of the universe, its specie ceased to be the consequence of a deliberate act of creation and, to make matters worse, its behaviour was governed not by reason but by involuntary and unconscious factors. But, the person, throw unarmed in this uncertain world, has the imperative need in believing in some protagonism of his own, even though it had no more that the consistency of a feather whipped by the gale.

What action of the new being could determine that its appearance took place on one continent or another, within a family in concord or another in continuous disagreement, in the midst of abundance or precariousness? How to reconcile this fact with the existence of freedom?

Certain psychic manifestations, such as obsessions, compulsions, phobias, and many others, all resulting from the struggle between opposing forces, reveal the absence of freedom and, of course, rule out the assertion that the person is governed by intelligence and reason, because many of these pictures are suffered by people of high level of reasoning. What is more, within this same context, it is unheard of to speak of will as one of the powers of the soul: a weapon useful only to deplete the vitality of the individual and channel his energies in a certain direction, in a so-called process of education, rather, it should be termed as a submission.

Therefore, if it is not possible to speak of freedom, it is hardly possible to speak of will, which would be the tool at the service of hypothetical freedom.

An action consequence of a free decision would finally be an act unmotivated and, therefore, placed outside the realm of rationality, which is the order in which we are accustomed to understand the events of life. For this reason we can't accept as compatible motivation and freedom. A purely free action would be a cause and never a consequence and would be outside the rational world. Why is it so pressing to decide whether or not free will exists? What would a world be like when this doubt did not arise? Is it, perhaps, to that world, without guilt, towards which mankind is directed?

The so-called mental illness would be proof, among many others, of the non-existence of human protagonism, so that it would be meaningless to speak of free will, neither could it be talk of guilt and the same would happen with the term responsibility. Consequently, moral judgment would be also meaningless.

## 5.3. Feminism

The relationship between men and women is frequently the subject of televised gatherings in which the opinions held lead to vehement discussions and bitter reproaches about the authorship of the couple's unhappiness. But I think that they are just the remnants of the eternal inclemency of life.

Except for pastime reasons, the wandering around the supremacy of one of the sexes over the other is a mere extravagance, so entering into this artificial contest, driven by resentment and not by the reason, is only the scene where to represent the grudges only attributable to the course of one's life. In addition, it supposes the neglect of the historical facts determining the evolution of both roles, because, in the end, someone had to abandon the protection of the cave to provide food for the offspring and someone, also, had to remain watching over the maintenance of the fire. Everyone has enough reasons to be upset by the harshness of life, but charging the bill for this disappointment on complementary sex can be, saving current circumstances in the coexistence of the couple, a mere relief but never a consistent deduction.

But, as Goytisolo's poetry says that "we are still on the road", such heated controversies may be the death throes for the complaint of living, until it is generalized the consideration that man and woman, hand in hand, have to be loyal friends in this difficult pilgrimage, putting, thus, an end to this sterile controversy.

Until that moment arrives, it seems that we are focused to live this debate as if we were followers of soccer equipment. In a publics manifestations, the head of one of the most powerful world powers declared himself to be a feminist, with a grave lack of knowledge of the limits of his representation, but this is one of the usual abuses of the political class that lives in the bubble of self-indulgence, of which it will not leave as long as their lives run through different channels than the rest of mortals, until they don't give up their irritating privileges, such as those of an early and generous retirement, the official cars, escorts, reserved parking spaces, special legal protections, and a number of privileges which, on the whole, foster the mistaken belief Of singularity that separates them from the rest of citizens whom they believe to serve.

## 5.4. The Past

Probably, for some matters it should be good that the past was only a corner where to keep the memories for to delight oneself or to mourn for them and that, in practical terms, they had not repercussions over the present, but this not the reality. The past is like a backpack, more or less heavy, in dependence with the lived experiences, from which the person can't be detached.

In the study of any evolutionary process one can't dispense with the knowledge of the past, as one can't calculate the length of a river without knowing the place of its birth. Surprisingly, which is common sense in any study, remains being a picturesque disquisition, for the Psychology. The application of psychological theories that take into account the past are considered impractical, as a mere waste of time. But reality is stubborn and does not bend to our desires. Current events, such as the endless political and other social struggles and the adoptions, are samples which serve to exemplify, as it could not be less, the importance of the past, both in the evolution of nations and in the behaviour of people.

The practical spirit, that characterizes the present life, considers the past a useless burden to bear, without realizing that the past, no matter what, is present and that it is not possible to scorn its constant and silent influence. After many years of the end of the Spanish civil war, there is still controversy about the authorship of the damage caused in it, as well as the judgment deserved by the contending sides and of its leaders. And, what could be even more striking, any parliamentary debate can lead to extemporaneous accusations. The fact that of the reference made to concrete events can't be inferred that they acquire full meaning disconnected from their precedents.

In the case that the reflection itself was not enough, the families that go to adoption can know of firsthand the decisive importance of the first years of life. When a family welcomes a child over the age of five, to put an age, they expect that the days with the new member go by in the same regularity as their lives did, and even how not to expect a certain trend to gratitude in consideration to the rescue of a dark future. But, which is the surprise when, after a very short honeymoon, the newcomer shows unexpected behaviour to soon start a rampant career that begins with visits to psychologists, subsequent reports to the police and income in special schools, in an endless calvary.

But, the behaviour does seem not to have sense, has it. The child is led by the same laws that govern the behaviour of all creatures who, after a brief adaptation to the new environment, return to the primitive path restoring to the new world all the frustrations and resentments accumulated in its first dates, which is not far from that which takes place after the honeymoon, when the lovers are faced with the triviality of daily life.

Nowadays, the theme of emigration and the problems that its reception arouses is a very pressing one. It is a problem that, rationally focused, should have an easy solution, taking into account the high level of development of western societies. But it is not so, and the explanation is simple because in this issue, as in most of that the existence poses, factors belonging to a field beyond the rational prevent the implementation of the appropriate plans. The mentioned factors are not superficial but sink their roots in a distant past. The education we have received and which, among others, is presided over by slogans as logical as that which says "wherever you go, do what you see", is impossible to comply for to all those people who, looking for protection and in our civilization. But we see, here again, how life, which has dispossessed all these people of any material good, has not been able, however, to detach them from their past.

The reckless disregard of past, generates these logical disenchantments.

## 5.5. The Self-Help manuals

Starting from the elementarily of the so-called best-seller-publications destined to the diffusion of the secrets of happiness-, it can soon be noticed that, although destined to promote well-being, they are in fact only correlates of the penances assigned to the old ones deviations from virtue after the pertinent confession, following the theory of kinship existing between current medicine and religious practice which, although it seems to be fighting retreat, still survives, disguised as science, in these supposed treaties of medicine.

Those known as self-help treatises are nothing more than a catalogue of councils whose following-up would have the same effect as the heavy armour to the weak warrior who, needing for his sustenance the remaining precarious energies, it would leave him prostrate before combat, achieving thus the opposite result to the promised one.

From my remembered teacher I heard, with surprise, that all writings have an advantage, even those full of follies. Such is the case of these widespread publications - very similar to the old sermons that, from the pulpit, showed us the path of sanctity- designed to teach us the procedures for achieving the well-being, as if it were a state that one could get through a few theoretical lessons.

It is worth paying attention to the paragraph of a widespread publication that affirms that "the means to achieve well-being are within the possibilities of each one of us. Personally, he continues, I think that a well-balanced combination of work, reflection and self-confidence are the ingredients needed to live an efficient life. I do not believe in naive formulas or historical excursions ... "Bravo! This is as much as affirming that it is convenient to bet on the precise number to be awarded with the lottery prize.

The belief that the person has the necessary devices to achieve an efficient life is, at least, objectionable. Let us see, if the person had on his hand the necessary weapons to not suffer, it would have to be concluded that the land would be populated by a group of idiots who suffer because they want it. No, things cannot be that simple. Moreover, defining what should be understood by efficient life is an unsuccessful task since each adjective would have to be defined with a new one which, in turn, would demand a new definition, in an endless adjustment work that would never achieve the objectives pursued.

In the previous paragraph it is stated not to believe in historical excursions, as if these were questions of faith, although it is true that this commentary expresses, at the same time, the disdain towards the Psychoanalysis; An absurd comment, because how to conjugate the transcendence of the childish events and that, at the same time, it is a waste of time to return on them to find there the causes of the current situation of the individual? For those who share the idea of the futility of the study of the past, I will say that only through it is it possible to access the knowledge of the person and, even more important, only with this knowledge can the person achieve his total acceptance and his inner friendship.

Self-help manuals, so fashionable today, are based on the naive belief that a person has the freedom to perform as many behavioral patterns were proposed, as if they could be regulated at will and could they be chosen, freely, among a varied repertoire of guidelines. This foolish believing is similar to the celebrated courses of Christianity, not too distant from today, in which the young men, even the most licentious of the community, underwent surprising transformations, passing from the shamelessness to the intolerance towards themselves and to the others, till they became a true sword of heretics and libertines. Fortunately, for the peace of the city, the change lasted like a summer storm and after a few days of being in a euphoric holiness, each one returned to where he used to. And it is that the behaviour is based on historical pillars, on rigid structures that hardly allow slight and provisional oscillations. The contrary it happens with the modifications derived from the knowledge based on the "insight" or internal perception.

It is said of self-help publications that give useful advice to better navigate through life. For example, if you leave the house and unexpectedly it starts to rain copiously, you have two options (really?): to get angry or taking it as something irremediable to get the best out of it. It is very simple, no? It is also said of the best thing for personal growth is to value oneself a lot. That is good, and how is it eaten?

Achieving well-being is a more complex matter than the simple drafting of a catalogue of recommendations. An agreement would not be reached to define what we understand for welfare, and yet in Psychology it has a very precise meaning, which is none other than the state of the person who is at peace with himself. But in order to reach this goal, one must first know one's self, an idea that is nothing new, for the same aphorism is already found in the temple frontispiece of Apollo, which translated into Latin comes to say "Gnosce te ipsum". Because, inviting a person to be positive sounds, at least, naive; The problem is how to do it. And if that was not enough, there it goes the consequent reflection: how is it that something so obvious and that would be of great benefit has not been put into practice before?

## 5.6. The Moral: The lie

The immediacy of daily communication requires the use of expressions that lack of psychological understanding, so many of the qualifiers that can serve as relief in daily life, have a different understanding in the field of Psychology. In general, any expression that has a moral connotation is opposed to the task of Psychology.

The set of passions, such as love, hatred, resentment, forgiveness, etc., omnipresent in the life of the people, with a clear moral connotation, lacks, however, of a psychological correlation. Colloquially the term will is used to emphasize how much a person can achieve by employing such a mysterious force. But in the light of judgment, and since liberty may be no more than a mirage, it would make no sense to believe in the existence of such power with which it is hoped to prevent the passions from overflowing.

Likewise, the term virtue which refers to the capacity for restraint of passion is equally a creation of human necessity in its attempt to put some order in anarchy. Therefore, virtue is a moral or social term but never a psychological one. The passions form an inseparable part of the instinctive equipment with which the person comes to the world, and the intensity of their manifestations is dependent on the conditions in which the being is going to develop, and their way of manifesting allows us to know how were his first steps in the world, just as the geologist can know the cataclysms of the past, with the simple study of the disposition of the geological strata.

Virtue is defined as the orientation towards the good. But, psychologically speaking, good coincides with inner peace or the absence of suffering. Also the virtues have been classified in the theological ones, which are infused by God in his creatures, and in the cardinal virtues; in none of them can a psychological correlate be found.

Leaving aside the faith, which is the result of an obliged and blind belief embodied in the process of education in a particular religious milieu, the hope is yet another example of what, despite being profusely employed and advised, lacks the psychological translation because, given the fact that the person hardly reaches his desires, it will have to be admitted that the hope is only an unsatisfied yearning, so that the positive thing in the life of the being is the hopelessness. Consequently, only after having passed through successive levels of anguish without succumbing, as Schopenhauer says, is it possible to achieve inner peace, the well-being that is installed in the person as a consequence of the denial of the will to live, which only differs from that advocated by Stoicism. Both orientations differ from the psychological point of view to which is just the flood of life that leads to get this goal, if it is ever reached. On the other hand, in following the guidelines of Stoicism up to the total renunciation of the satisfaction of desires, as well as in the achievement of the denial of the will to live, neither reason nor the enigmatic will serve as utensils. For the psychological approach only the initial conditions determines the degree of coexistence with despair.

The same will be said of the so-called vices and their

lack of psychological significance. For example, without the existence of selfishness, understood as an instinctive faculty of dealing with material and spiritual survival, the being would perish. For the psychological understanding, egoism is, apart from being inseparable from the being, its protector. Different is what happens in the field of social morality that understands it as the incarnation of evil.

It is wrong to refer to anyone as an angry person because, in doing so, it generalizes what is only a circumstantial trait, what would be the anger that invades a person at a given moment. Equally unfortunate is to say that someone is vengeful because in this case the reference is not made to the essence of the person but to his circumstance, because revenge, another instinct that enjoys a bad fame but that, no matter what, is simply the instinctive response to the outrage received by which discharge, prompt or delayed, the psychic apparatus achieves some relief.

All these comments are summarized in the reflection that the so-called theological virtues, as the cardinal ones, prudence, justice, strength and temperance, are not capacities that the person can voluntarily exercise, because these are the product of the interaction of external factors beyond to its decision. It will be said that this is a pessimistic view of the existence and the denial of any role of the person, but mediating in this debate is not the object of these comments. In addition, we would be in the same circle in which being pessimistic or optimistic is no option at all; Life is, finally, a mixture of illusion and discouragement. Do not forget that everything here is referred to the psychological side of knowledge and in its name cannot be confused the desires and the realities, what we like and what bothers us.

Probably the most unjust offense is to equate the lies and the wickedness because whoever is forced to lie, just pay the tribute imposed by the dominant to the subordinate. It is for this reason that the lie is more an inescapable necessity than a moral transgression; it is the result of a tyrannical dependence. For if the person were certainly free, he would never accept the overload that the lie entails for the psychic apparatus, since it obliges us to remember the data of omission so as not to be caught in contradiction. Do not to be able of avoiding to lie is the same as to have to suffer a damage in the psychic instance of the self because when you lie, you must be careful to remember the falsified data which, in turn, requires the sequestration of a quantity of memory that, thus, remains outside of the free disposition. The lie takes place, not because the person is morally dubious, but whenever the truth clashes with insurmountable fears. Where is, then, the benefit of the transgression that could deserve our condemnation?

Of course, the lie would never occur without the existence of a censorship of impossible avoidance, nor would the Shrovetide have taken place if the customs had been more permissive throughout the year.

## 5.7. Urbanism and Housing

Psychology, while aiming to offer an understanding of the person as a previous condition to the establishment of an inner harmony, must also take into account the environmental conditions that surround its development; Otherwise its value would be scarce.

A long time ago, our political representatives determined that vertical construction was the best option for the development of our cities which, although having its advantages, seems the least appropriate model for the favourable development of the family since to live within a rickety space with frequent absence of visual horizon and the scarcity of space make, the habitat an ideal medium for that the logical tensions of coexistence to rebound between its nearby walls without finding drainage. Having so much space, it is already sad that society has found this subterfuge, more convenient for abuse and corruption in the adjudication of building land than for the development of the childhood.

The physical frame of the home is the space in which most of a person's life runs, from childhood to the end of life. Yet our architects and town planners design homes and cities without consideration all this factors. Fortunately, the technological advance allows the homes to be emancipated from environmental rigors that, in a near past, advised the construction of cramped buildings. Neither is distance the obstacle of then. There is no reason, therefore, to continue on the same path.

The amplitude of spaces is determinant in the development of the person; Just look at the jubilation with which the children and the puppies contemplating the preparations before going out into the street. Deepness of horizons and good thermal and acoustic insulation are physical aspects of housing whose importance is idle to point out.

Also is worthy to put attention the importance that, when senescence arrives, the person does not have to change of the house and can be protected by the same reference points that framed the days of his existence, because when lost those points of orientation, the confusion rushes dizzily.

## 5.8. Health

The concern for eternal salvation, which until recently claimed so many sacrifices and efforts, has now been replaced by meticulous health care that demands no less vigilance and solicitude. The efforts that were once devoted to the salvation of souls today find their correspondence in the effort to maintain health. The reduction of the time of stay in the purgatory, that once was achieved through the accumulation of plenary indulgences, today you get the same through the repeated explorations, analyzes and prescriptions. Likewise, cathedrals and parishes have their substitutes in the gigantic hospitals and dispensaries. Also the book of saints has its replica in the innumerable days destined to (celebrate?) the different diseases; thus, we have the day of cancer, the day of the heart, of the diabetes, etc.

The same diligence that was dispensed in the conquest of eternal salvation, unfolds, in our days, in the attainment of a healthy state. And as in the pursuit of that purpose there could be no weakness or hesitation, for salvation could be lost with the slightest scorn, the same attention must be paid to health, for those who hesitate in the strict observance of the meticulous catalogue of patterns conducive to attaining a healthy life, could be precipitated to the hell of the disease.

Thus, the dentist demands a daily cleaning of not less than ten minutes; The proctologist a biannual review, at least; The gynaecologist advises a periodic examination of the breasts; The otolaryngologist requests regular inspection of the hearing apparatus; The ophthalmologist, that of the vision; The urologist does not renounce his assignment and threatens to require a regular prostate examination, starting at a certain age; The osteopath advises the tracing of the locomotors apparatus and measurement of bone mass.

Neither, the general medical practitioner, wants to be left behind in this frantic career and periodically remembers the obligation to measure the levels of glucose, folic acid, etc. Particularly intense has been the campaign to contain the levels of cholesterol, a perverse element until some kindly researchers rescued a mode of nice cholesterol from purgatory, arriving at the temerity, even, of saying that atherosclerosis is independent of the accumulation of cholesterol In blood. No one knows, because heretics have always existed. What is certain is that the measurement of a myriad of parameters makes health care almost an illness.

The fulfillment of this new zeal has benefited from the massive desertion of temples and the accommodation in new places of worship, such as outpatient clinics and hospitals, with serious disruption to the public coffers that tread inexorably towards ruin. But, as already happened with the religious matters, here the passionate suffocates all possible criticism.

And so, in this new cult, there are curious phenomena such as the growing opinion that has led to consider the sun, our faithful giver of life and light, as one of the most traitors enemies of humanity of which we must defend with a big variety of creams and protections, because the dermatologist warns of the advent of terrible evils for those who dare to receive it without the pertinent caution. Thus, we contemplate how in the pools and beaches children and adults face the sun covered in dresses.

News of surprising discoveries, that promise an imminent return to youth appear daily in newspapers, almost always coming from America. The new products that stop the passage of the time (anti-aging products) invade the advertising spaces. Eye drops, creams for muscle pain, collagen to prevent joint wear and an endless number of remedies whose observance it would require, at least, twenty-four hours a day, leaving the person with no time to live. And, as it could not be otherwise, we have the same ingenuity than the children and believe that "what you eat is what you manufacture". And it is by virtue of this belief that sharks are bound to be paralytic, since the consumption of their cartilage It's destined to alleviate the effects of age. The regular practice of sport has become an obsessive penance. And in this context, the lives of people are framed by a number of warnings without review. Thus, although no one has provided any evidence, the paranormal phenomena are still in force as they also continue to come on the market prepared to combat alopecia.

The maintenance of health requires, in addition, a careful care of the food and, parallel to the happened with the sex, also here it is necessary "to learn to feed" for whose teaching has appeared the figure of the nutritionist at the same time that in television are trendy the cooking's programs, which show the incessant are y touching of food until it is left arranged in surprising forms, probably destined more to the liking of the eyes than to the taste of the palate.

Naturism and its derivatives, like veganism, preach the return to the times in which pests were fed on the scarce food. And it is that, like historically has been happening, assimilating abundance is a subject little less than impossible, as well as digesting success. We live in permanent protest against the progress made from the caverns and in the exaltation of the its inexplicable benefits of the past days, when the person was exposed to such a critical conditions like the uncertainty of leaving the cave without guarantees of return, the rigors of the life in the open air, the plagues and the hunger. But it seems that the plethora of food in our supermarkets is revitalizing the everlasting feeling of guilt, because this is the only way to understand the cult of ecology, naturism, veganism and so many other movements that share the longing for a frightening past.

In the face of such confusion, the timely question is whether it is worth keeping health at such a high price.

One of the hypotheses to explain this state of affairs is that the human being, tired of its insignificance, reacts with the haughtiness proportional to the submission undergone for millennia and has come to think himself domineering the functioning of life and the laws that govern the march of our planet and, thus, begins to dream of dominating the universe. It may be that, with that pride, it is believed with the right to dictate, as the religious shepherds did, the norms that govern the functioning of the individual life.

Thus, the permanence in the youth and freshness demands great efforts. At the beginning of Christmas, the television spaces are populated with advertisements for cosmetics that bring us back to the youth. Few comments deserve the thousands of instruments that will avoid the undesirable consequences of the passage of days, such as those intended to solve the problem of tired legs of the elderly, who end up exhausted by tortuous exercises.

The pretension to establish a rigor in the practice of medicine, and in general in any profession, is as much as having a naive view of things, a lack of knowledge of the multitude of factors and commitments that surround existence. In this respect it is thought that in the same way that the function shapes the organ, it demands its function. Recently, in an absurd journalistic article, certain laboratories were blamed for "creating" diseases to seek their remedies. But let's take a simple example: if a diagnostic centre, equipped with very expensive material, is opened, who will not doubt that the prescription of certain tests, other than the diagnostic value sought, could be related to the need to pay off such investment?

If the passage of days has been obstructing the channel through which the torrent of religion flows, it is consequent to think that its waters have sought new channels and, in this sense, it may be that medicine is replacing its ancestral importance, since the helplessness of being somewhere will have to find relief and probably the current cult of health be the new channel.

However, the necessary requisite for this obsessive devotion to health to be installed, with such strong rooting, goes through the assumption that the natural state of the person is that of the disease, as in the past the imploring plea for forgiveness was based

Under this exaltation for health, the so-called preventive medicine is experiencing an unprecedented boom and society runs wit frenzy behind the holy water of explorations and drugs that will avoid all ills. The same course that followed the religion I am afraid that is going through the preventive medicine: first it was decided that the cholesterol was essentially harmful to rescue soon a good variety of it, as already was done with the angels and the demons, on the conviction that sin flooded the whole life.

The advertising spaces of television are populated with ads that promise to maintain the juvenile skin aspect in such a way like if the time were no passing, leaving no trace whatsoever. Also, the publicity of a battalion of laxatives comes to us to say that the intestinal movement, essentially reflex, has lost the memory and has to be taught. Within this framework of the senseless resistance to the inevitable aging, the laboratories have put their sights on a factor that inevitably accompanies it, which is the deterioration of the joints and, thus, is in a position to decree that collagen is the substance of modern communion.

While all these follies take place, the modern inquisition makes a new index of prohibited products, among which one of the most pernicious matters is the white sugar. The milk is also in the inquisitorial point of look, and it's difficult that obtains the approval if it has not previously been dislodged from the noxious lactose. And so the caffeine is removed from the coffee, the bread without gluten, and all food will finally be light. A day will come on which even the spermatozoids of the seminal fluid are excluded.

Here is the paradox: on the one hand, the pride and on the other, the pessimism that prevents the enjoyment for what has been achieved. There are superb documentaries about nature whose portentous images we could enjoy on the formidable screens of our televisions, if not were for the apocalyptic words with which they unfailingly conclude: unfortunately the excessive ambition of the unscrupulous companies puts -to the particular species of the documentary film, in each case- on the verge of extinction.

## 5.9. Pessimism and Arrogance

The set of fears associated with modern acquisitions, such as the waves of mobile telephony, transgenic foods, etc., are updates of the everlasting fears that the human race has been suffering since its inception. These misgivings are part of the paradoxical behaviour of the person who, on the one hand, recognizes himself defenceless and on the other, feels with the necessary power to compromise the survival of our planet. An arrogant presumption thinking that the human race could destroy something so great. In this scen, the environmentalists are the transcription of itinerant preachers of the recent past, ready to alert the consciences and awaken culpability before the imminent arrival of the end of the world.

The undeniable advances in industrialization, communication and robotics, to name a few examples, intimidate man greatly and force him to question whether, after what has such a promising aspect, a catastrophe will not be hidden. Pleasure and sin continue to be chained, preventing the enjoyment of the advantages that the times have brought.

The increase in food production, which should reassure the inhabitants of more developed societies, is, on the contrary, a source of torture, probably aroused by the feeling of guilt implicit in the false belief in a rebellion against biblical condemnation.

If you can cover considerable distances in a comfortable cockpit equipped with climate control, listening to the favourite music and helped of a pilot who leads us safely to unknown destinations, a hidden voice will be alerted that will reproach us for melting the Arctic; If, looking at the exuberant supermarkets full of exotic products, the same impertinent voice will censure us to be rusting the earth and will urge us to embrace "veganism", naturism or any kind of sects that preach the return to nature, to the Emilio, whose author, by the way, was depositing his five children in an orphanage as they were being born.

This extemporaneous behaviour brings to my memory the surprising observation I heard from my beloved teacher, Dr. Molina: "Success is very difficult to assimilate". For spectacular the conquests may be, he will always be at the man's back, like a contumacious shadow, the voice that brings him out of joy and turns pride into the signal of the advent of a new disaster. All progress is the emissary of a fatal tragedy, before which there will be no better amulet than penance and renunciation, since mankind has inside his soul that the evils of the earth will always be due to his bad behaviour.

Ignorance, fanaticism, and arrogance seem to have allied themselves to obscure human contentment by their conquests. At every step it stirs the never-dormant consciousness that affea all our actions and does make us feel guilty of all beneficial modification. To such a point arrives his irritability that we, poor of us!, are considered the actors of a hypothetical destruction of the planet and, because of it, we are pushed to repentance, to return to the caves and to the solemn crusade for the salvation of the planet that, poor of we!, only in our dreams we could put in danger.

This unusual arrogance appeared on the occasion of the discovery of a supposed hole in the ozone layer. And although the human eye has only been contemplating the earth for two days from outer space, it was no obstacle to make as many conjectures as possible to exalt this dark spirit. And so the candid chlorofluorocarbon compounds began to nourish the catalogue of malefic agents.

But nothing new is here because throughout history every infrequent phenomenon has been interpreted as the prelude to the end of the world to which the celebrated Nostradamus set a date, as did the Mayans, although the latter, having established a closer term, have fallen into discredit.

The haughtiness of our days, which flies freely in the wings of the nonsense, without the slightest sense of ridicule, accuses us of "destroying the planet" and, consequently of this, the birth of the "progressive" movement offered for the redemption, inviting us to "to save the planet". And in these we are.

Sins against the environment have replaced the ancestral ones of the flesh. The so-called greenhouse effect, which is not well known if it will conclude with the freezing of the planet or with the increase in temperature that melts the polar masses and causes the immersion of extensive terrestrial zones, is one of the phrases that we repeat as parrots.

## 5.10. The History

The essays on history suffer from the vices, peculiar to Psychology and Philosophy, because most of them try to accommodate the facts to the desires, something like conclusions to the menu. The facts are hardly taken into account as such, in their fatal reality, but there is always, the more or less concealed, an insinuation that the consequences may have been different from how they have been presented with only the variation of some small circumstance. It is common to hear that the appearance of this or that celebrity changed the course of history, when it seems more accurate to think that the appearance of such a person was, in turn, the consequence of latent conditions, in the same way as in a determined moment the water solidifies itself due to the previous descents of temperature, not by its exposure to the cold in the last minute or as who, drunk, attributes its state to the last glass.

As happens in any discipline in which the purpose pursued is the understanding, the facts of history, whether we like it or not, are immovable, so it is not coherent to be upset because a general lost a battle or because Hannibal, at the same gates of Rome, did not decided to take it. Trying to make the data fit a given ideology is the widespread misunderstanding in our days. No, history follows a course that escapes all our expectations and sympathies and, as in Psychology, its study can help to understand the past but not to predict the future, not even which way would be the most successful to follow.

As has been commented, the studies of history keep a clear parallel with the psychiatric practice. To the consultation come people exposing facts, immovable by definition, which constitute the reason of the consultation itself. However, all too often it occurs here as with the exposition of historical facts, which are hardly accepted as such, and are frequently rejected with the same puerile argument that if so-and-so had not acted in this way the story would have changed his course and the deplorable consequences would not have been deduced. But these infantile outbursts, unfit for any intellectual exercise, have nothing to do with the study of history, which is moved by the unfathomable compendium of the passions of its characters whose purpose, if any, escapes the human understanding.

## 5.11. Psychology and Philosophy

The confusion of the terms "to be" and "to stay" is a frequent failure of the understanding of the person that, in short, is the exclusive purpose of Psychology.

In a colloquial communication, the application to a person of a certain moral qualifier, may be due to a tolerable relief and to lack, therefore, of greater transcendence, nor would the misspellings in a writing destined to end up in the trash can; But when is to be presented to an important examination or, if it is appropriate to understand a situation of a person, the incorrectness can be striking.

The term being is always referred to the essence of

the person and, on the contrary, the term to stay is the resultant set of the action modelling the circumstances. When it is affirmed that Angel is ordained, we speak improperly since a quality is attributed to him that in no way corresponds to the essence of his person and yes to his circumstances, since, as far as the being is concerned, we all come in the same way to the world: naked of material and spiritual clothing. So it is, that many thinkers, considering the reference to being as an individual entity to be insufficient, have found necessary to include other additions Such is the case of the existentialist school, which in speaking of being does it as an entity inseparably linked to the world, resulting that the definition of being is the synthesis of being in the world with others. In a similar way, our great thinker Ortega and Gasset in his eloquent manifestation: I am myself and my circumstances, manifesting with it the idea that we are something more than individual beings, we are living beings in continuous modelling by the influence of the others and of the environment, a factor that will finally explain the peculiar characteristics of being in the world.

At the beginning, the being is only an instinctive equipment searching for satisfying the need and in that eagerness there is no distinction between the ones and the others; Is the unequal way in which particular circumstances affect the growth process from which the particular position of his being will be deduced. Circumstances behave similarly to what the theatre director does before beginning the rehearsals of a new play: sharing the roles of the play. For this reason, it is not an original idea to equate life with a great theatrical performance in which each plays the assigned role. In the case of the theatre director there is a certain decision in the cast; Not so in the actors for whom the role is imposed.

This lack of discernment between these two concepts is the origin of misunderstandings, if not of reproaches and even insults, such as can be received by clients of certain psychiatrists obsessed to obtain practical results through the use of guidelines and advices. Working thus, it happens that before the third visit, the client results being the responsible for an evolution below the psychiatrist's expectations. Let us take a very frequent example in which a person returns home, again and again, to make sure that the key of the gas has been conveniently closed. Does the psychiatrist think that the person suffering such an ordeal is not aware of irrationality of his procedure, as to receive instructions on how to close the key? In this case he would be better to be advised by a locksmith; at least it would not be confused or censored. This always happens whenever the psychiatrist forgets that the client comes to understand the enigma that underlies in so tortuous going and returning and that it is the simplification of more extensive fears, which cover the whole life of the individual.

If the Psychiatry aspires to be a science, it must leave the modifying spirit, that misunderstanding practical sense that, in any case, would be more appropriate for the profession of mechanic. Moreover, Psychiatry is a discipline full of simplicity, contrary to the idea that people has. It only has to subject to the purpose of understanding through deduction, extracting the consequences of facts proposed by the formulation of simple hypotheses; everything else is banality, presumption, arrogance or eagerness to dominate, everything less than a scientific procedure. And for this, we must start at the principle: listen to the story of who comes, who in no way does it in the search for advice or guidelines to avoid what makes you suffer; He does so only in the hope of finding someone with whom he can decipher the enigma that contains the apparent nonsense of what causes him uneasiness.

In any case, we may be at the beginning of a stage in which Psychiatry finally opts for the path of knowledge, unravelling the rich symbolic content of spiritual symptoms, leaving for other specialties the organic explanations and away from the traditional and empty rhetoric. In this regard, I recall the performance of a celebrated professor whose clinical sessions were spent asking to the pupils about the diagnosis of the clinical case presented, while objecting to how many opinions responded to his incessant interpellations. Something should have heard about the procedure used by Socrates, the maieutic dialogue, although unlike the famous philosopher, he did not pretend that the students would find into themselves the solution, but highlight his supposed wisdom. In short, it was the simple stratagem of taking a detail for the whole, as if putting the fingers on the keyboard of the piano were enough for to believe that one is an accomplished pianist.

## 5.12. Frequent Errors of Psychiatric Terminology

Without losing sight of the procedural nature of life, we will understand that many of the expressions used in the field of Psychology have no appropriate meaning. For example, recovery is an inaccurate expression because it refers to the return to an earlier state, as if it were a flu process. Spiritual suffering always comes from the early days of life, although they can manifest more openly for external observation, but not for those who suffer them.

In the same way, it must be understood that the use of the expression rehabilitate, apart from being in itself inadequate, the more proper application to behaviours that after a period of delirium return to the fold of social coexistence, does not translate any psychological reality, because the sense here is ethical but nothing adds to the psychological understanding.

Likewise, in situations in which the person has interrupted a period of dependency, the only thing that has changed is the outside because in relation to the basic situation that led to seek relief in another more tolerable reality remains intact, unless they have lived extraordinary experiences.

Another reproach that can be made to the current exercise of Psychology is its mechanistic orientation. Thus, the client is often advised to develop strategies and skills to deal with the evil that afflicts him, which, apart from being an insult to his intelligence, is an unnecessary task, as with all advice.

We live in the epidemic of "masters" and it is no surprise that they have been programmed for the most varied destinations, such as the "master's degree in family management" or "expertise in duel management". In short, everything is treated as if it were a war or a police tactic destined to solve a crime.

We shall conclude that many of the psychological explanations are accepted without taking into account the serious absurdity of their propositions; perhaps the need is responsible for the absence of criticism, as in the past happened with religious sermons. It is not uncommon to hear from the mouths of psychologists such pious statements that the suffering of the client is due to the overprotection from their parents, without any criticism that protection can never be excessive, because when it seems so, we would have to speak of selfishness at the not allowing the other person to live the experiences that life brings.

## 5.13. The Function of Fantasy

In the realm of spiritual sufferings, fantasy is still regarded as an idle guest, only useful in bringing about damages to the people that they abandon themselves to it. From this point of view we must accept that we are still under the influence of the religious currents that contemplate life as a delicate crossing at the mercy of multiple temptations of devastating effects among which, due to its extraordinary virulence, highlights leisure. It is not uncommon, therefore, that, starting from the observation that in many spiritual sufferings there is an exacerbation of the imaginative capacity, its creation is imputed to it, ignoring that it is only its inevitable consequence. To combat thus the fantasy, which is nothing but the shield and relief of the unbearable torment of existence, is like taking the radish for the leaves, the effects by its causes. What is the Psychologist's mission is the searching for coherence that exists behind the fantastic creation.

Identical protective function has the dream production. Thus, when the mother, whom the son commits suicide after an endless string of violent incidents that ended with his expulsion from the home, dreams that he returns, knocking at the door, trying to open it with a different key, until she joyfully welcomes him to the entrance, while greeting him affectionately and welcoming him with an unprecedented tenderness, she carries out the most profound of her wishes.

The fantasy has, therefore, a foundation and an undeniable utility. From the unrepeatable times of "Peña Retama" I remember how the obstinate argumentative persecution to a delirious development concluded in an attempt of suicide.

In short, Psychology and Psychiatry should understand that the suffering is not due from an excessive production of fantasy, but that is the shelter where the person seeks protection, as the sailboat whipped by the storm of the sea, seeks the harbour. If we do not change the present state of things, we may affirm that, although the psychiatric conceptions are impregnated with the religious spirit, temptation and sin, the so-called therapies based on admonition and advice are, in its turn, contaminated by the idea of miracle.

The purpose of fantasy is to attend the interests of the individual, serving as a counterweight to the frustration inherent in the state of helplessness of the living being, a characteristic feature of existence. Thanks to the conscious fantasy, the person is able to modify the world, to live new lives, to embody characters of fiction, to recreate comfortable situations and to anticipate another's feared, thus alleviating the unbearable weight of the lack of protection. In this dilemma, dreams and fantasies are to the psychic apparatus what the vitamins to the body: essential elements for its more adequate functioning.

Hence, the critical logic towards a particular care, psychiatric and psychological, based on the effort to combat, at any price and without respite, the production of fantasy as the promoter of the most undesirable mental manifestations, instead of the obligatory dedication of to unravel their meaning. At this point I feel like a one of the heretics, opposed to such an extended endeavour.

Psychiatry, which, as a practical discipline, deals with the improperly called psychic disease and which aspires to correct its manifestations, the symptoms, without first having reached an understanding of them, tends to proclaim that the imaginative function is what causes the "illness". Thus, guided by the delusional stories offered by people who have suffered acute psychotic outbreaks, one would have the temptation to believe that fantastic creation is to the prone person what the proximity of the heroin to the drug addict. Pictures such as schizophrenia, acute psychotic outbreaks, obsessive states, etc. are thought to be propitiated by abusive complacency in fantastic, which would inexorably lead to their addiction. To this conclusion one arrives confusing the causes with the effects and vice versa. Such a mistake would not occur if occasionally we were to consider that the refuge in fantasy is the natural counterweight of a life, fundamentally, dominated by the uncertainty, or its referents: helplessness and fear. Because existence is a huge market in which only occasionally we carry out a satisfactory transaction and that, when this happens exceptionally its effects are so ephemeral that, in the face of such a gloomy panorama, it is necessary to resort to fantastic creation, to refuge in the imagination. It could be that fantasy was the only form of freedom that the individual knows. That is why, what concerns to the purpose of the imaginative function is what should deserve the most interest.

## 5.14. The Memory

Pushing the memory, the ability to store and rescue information is the interest that can be spontaneous or forced. The Images, whether mental, visual or auditory, are stored in the physical support of nervous tissue of capacity, although immense, limited. The sentence that says that knowledge occupies no place seems not to be confirmed. Possibly to save some data, we must get rid of another's.

There is a portion of memory ready to be rescued at will, memory that we could call of the free access, and another that is not at our disposal but that can show its content at the least expected moment.

The recording of the scenes that will nourish the flow of memories will be all the more firm with the more emotional charge are, the earlier they have been lived and the more t It often happens that in complaints about loss of memory, what fails is the existence of a real interest in remembering, however consciously the person is convinced otherwise. Therefore, when someone complains about losing memory, it must be taken into account that the memory is never lost, simply the rescue of it may not be available at the desired time. They attend to the being of oneself, next to the personal interests.

It often happens that in complaints about loss of memory, what fails is the existence of a real interest in remembering, however consciously the person is convinced otherwise. Therefore, when someone complains about losing memory, it must be taken into account that memory never it's lost, simply the rescue of it may not be available at the desired time.

Going through carefully the pages of the life of people who, in the words of many frivolous thinkers, end in different forms of spiritual suffering in which the complain is the difficulty of remembering, one has the impression that they are beings that have simply spent their lives satisfying others' ambitions, being mere incarnations of a strange aspirations, spokesmen for other longings; serving, in short, to foreign purposes. They are people to whom the life has not authorized to approach to the care of themselves, in such a way that the final stage of their lives surprises them without any patrimony with which to entertain their thoughts since the memories, even being their own, are equally impregnated with this lack of protagonism. The life of these people is comparable to the trip that is made in the midst of the fog and apathy, which will scarcely leave memories. In any case, when someone complains of losing memory, he betrays himself at the very moment that remembers what he misses. These complaints are frequent are frequent at the beginning of old age, when life no longer offers any novelty.

The intensity of the fixation of the memories is related to the level of interest with which the successive events have been lived and this, in its turn, will be directly proportional to the degree of protagonism had in them. The presence of the person in the episodes of his life is the condition to satisfy his natural curiosity and to be able to incorporate the valuable elements to the personal patrimony that will form a treasure for when, in the last section of life, the news are scarce and intensified the dialogue to which Antonio Machado refers to when he writes: “I talk to the man who always goes with me”. Only then will a friendly interlocutor be available.

It is more than probable that if the person were protagonist of the passages of his life it would not be possible to suffer the picture baptized by Alzheimer, nor, it would produce the loss of memory, because in relation to this the organism behaves with it in a similar way as the computer does with the hard disk. The information is saved, without loss, ready to be rescued upon request. No memory is lost, only the interest.

It is attributed to the Alzheimer's picture, in addition to the behavioral manifestations of dementia, the loss of memory of recent events, a complaint frequently also expressed by other people in the absence of any alteration. It must be taken into account that the life cycle, both physical and psychic, is naturally governed successively by processes of assimilation and catabolism. In this, it is comparable to the curve described by an object thrown into space, which rises up to the zenith and from which begins an irreversible fall until it encounters the ground.

The combination of these two factors: the anabolism, that governs the first part of life, and the subsequent catabolism, together with the intensity of the person's participation in their experiences, would serve not to need to search for neurological alterations such like the neuronal atrophy or the existence of senile plaques in explaining the aetiology of Alzheimer's disease, In fact, it participates in the same course as the general aging in which the interest in the surrounding world decreases, day by day, although here, in addition to being earlier that the first neurological manifestations, is preceded by a more precarious life course than in the generality of the people.

If you reflect on the obsessive suffering, soon, we will realize that we have all had a similar episode although its duration and intensity have been of a lower degree, which allows the deduction that all, to a greater or lesser extent, we participate in the same universal happen. It would be the same as in other psychological manifestations, such as delusions. Whoever hears a delirious account, and has a minimum degree of empathy, will easily relate the incongruity of the narrative to the manifest content of dreams. Such is the likeness, that delirium is known as the dream of the awake up people.

In my opinion, the Alzheimer's illness is a mode of existence, it is the consequence of a life spent in the neglect of one's own interests, so that once it is manifest, it is not possible to alter its course or, much less, the finding of curative drugs since there is something that is absolutely refractory to any modification; that is, simply, the past. There is a date, in the calendar of health, dedicated to Alzheimer's disease, I do not know if for to celebrate its presence or to fight against it. The daring comes to the point of talking about prevention, but its disappearance will not be produced by any pharmacological discovery but, like everything else, because the advancement of the living conditions makes impossible his existence. In any case there are already on the market drugs that promise the restitution of memory loss or containment of their decline.

I have always wondered if it is humanitarian to submit these unfortunate beings to the tortuous exercises of inserting a ring in a circle of the same colour or the square in its corresponding place. Perhaps there is no answer to this question and the only answer will be, as always, in the imposition of one's life whose laws we do not know. In any case, as in the matter of the "restlessness" any movement will have to be done, everything but not stay still.

## 5.15. Loneliness

Is widespread the idea that lack of companionship and solitude is the same thing, and it may be for any observer, but in psychological terms the concept of solitude has a different meaning.

Let us see, even in the absence of an interlocutor, the person maintains a permanent dialogue with the internal instance that we have called the superego, or moral conscience, a dialogue particularly manifest in the resting hour, when, on the pillow, one reviews the actions of the day, which extend in the memories of past times, till the dream invades the conscious activity.

This intimate conversation can be as varied as varied are the various ingredients present in the formation of moral consciousness. This explains the fact that in some cases this conversation is presided over by friendship, and in others, however, by the incessant interpellation and contempt, in endless gradations. Well, in a psychological sense, loneliness is the lack of company or the bad company of one with oneself.

Those who have the truth that loneliness is the state of the persons separated from the others that keep in mind that in solitude one is born and in his company walks through the moors of life until with it is reached the inn of the last dream. Loneliness is always our company. There is no pain or sorrow that others may suffer for us, nor joys that can be shared with our own intensity.

From what has been said, it follows that, for Psychology, the term welfare, which in no way refers to the present environmental conditions, must be understood as a "being well with oneself", in the absence of internal conflicts or as a state of relationship cordial between the psychic instances of ego and superego. Therefore, it is an outrage to infer that due to environmental changes a person may suffer mental suffering susceptible to psychiatric care. It is necessary to distinguish the environmental alterations of the ailments to which we have been referring. It is one thing to not be at peace with oneself and another very different is to suffer the consequences of a catastrophe, like the loss of a loved one. Achieving this well-being is not the result of voluntary effort or follow-up of any pattern; it is something inherited as an immaterial good from the thresholds of life.

The possession of this well-being is projected in all the activities without needing to obtain notoriety or applause. The person is well paid with only the satisfaction that comes with good work, which is the same as "being oneself". But, to reaches this, the life has had to have been generous, it has had to allow that the desperation has not stopped, like storm, the genuine aspirations; that the doubt does not provoke startles; that the provisional nature and the relativity of the efforts do not cause uneasiness; that the course of days consents to the establishment of a serene scepticism; that the possession of some stoicism in the government of desires confers serenity and, finally, that the passage of the leaves of the calendar authorizes to enjoy this solitude in such good company.

Then - and here comes the annoying question - can not the person do nothing, so capable of inventing machines that substitute physical effort and provide us with homes so far from the caves of our dawn? Well, the answer is that nothing can be done, except represent the assigned role. And then, what is Psychology for? For something extremely important: to allow the person to be aware that life is a unbroken chain of their moments, preventing, thus, the irrational feelings of strangeness and guilt from disturbing the friendly relationship that must preside over the aforementioned intimate dialogue.

## 6. CURRENT DISEASES

One of the requirements of science is the achievement of an explanation that covers as many phenomena as possible. Well, here we have a new sample of the opposite: the accumulation of many names to describe states that have the same explanation and all this covered in the fact that by disease is no longer understood only well defined and static entities, such as happened in my years of faculty, but its significance has spread, accepting any alteration, more or less serious, of health; any variation, both physical and spiritual, may deserve the term disease, to the surprise of those who are finishing the practice of medicine.

One of the possible interpretations for this fact is that the current generation does not resign to the role of a simple companion and wants to "describe" new cadres, as did doctors of the past generations or naturists when contemplating the shape of a leaf not yet registered in the inventory. Perhaps, they are remnants of the nostalgia of the golden age of science.

The following are examples of this descriptive fever and, perhaps, of the striving for notoriety of many of its "discoverers" and, at the same time, testimonies of the enormous social advance by the fact to take into account complaints traditionally despised by its presentation near to the facts of everyday life.

## a) Fibromyalgia

Whenever a set of symptoms were resistant to how many therapies were prescribed, the problem was solved affirming that it was a rebellious picture to the treatment or was baptized with the name of neurasthenia. Of recent incorporation in the medical inventory, the so-called Fibromyalgia is an example of diffuse ailments that contravene all medical precautions. It is, at the same time, a sample of how medicine works when it is into perplexity.

Fibromyalgia is a confusing picture that can harbour a whole series of dispersed manifestations that, until recent times, were encompassed in the term neurasthenia; A picture characterized by an invincible fatigue, along with other painful manifestations that converge in a continuous complaint. But, as is so often the case today, this whole set of erratic complaints had to have a framework, correspond to an entity, and thus the term Fibromyalgia was born which, like a tailor's box, accommodates how many undisciplined manifestations come from the lips of the customers.

The coining of the term Fibromyalgia is the attempt to bring order to the anarchy of symptoms. Firstly the name of Fibrositis, or Psychogenic Rheumatism, was proposed to mean that the manifestations appeared in very particular personalities until, recently, this group of evanescent complaints was baptized like Fibromyalgia and, as such, accepted today by the World Health Organization.

To comment this, like other entities of recent baptism, we must take into account the simplicity of the mechanism used: simply to move the expressions of the client to the inventory of diseases. This is how we are surprised to find a number of new ailments.

Because, despite the mathematical character that is aspired to give to the medical knowledge, there is an insurmountable obstacle that is the subjectivity of the symptom. How to evaluate the pain that a person says to suffer, if much or little, excessive or restrained? All this difficulty, also, has economic and legislative repercussions, in that it promotes the start of expensive tests as well as legislative changes, frequently lacking in rigor.

But it seems that many of the people with this unclassifiable pain and such a discomfort have found peace once they have finally been sheltered in the diagnosis of Fibromyalgia

### b) Bulling

This name is intended to describe situations of harassment in which the victim is persecuted and intimidated, bringing, as a consequence of the repeated incidence, a decrease in the self-esteem of the victim. This is how it is described, although the self-esteem can't be entirely attributed to a specific circumstance since, as has been said, it is the result of a whole succession of historical circumstances, being the earliest the ones of the greatest repercussion.

These situations of abuse are not at all new and it is doubtful that they deserve a particular chapter in medical descriptions and not in the school system. In any case, and guided by what is stated in previous pages, it must be repeated that the configuration of one's own esteem takes place within the family frame and from the moment the new being appears in life. The rest can add or subtract more damage but never be the only cause.

### c) Burnout

Another picture recently incorporated in the psychiatric vademecum is the one known by the term Burnout, also denominated Working Syndrome or to be burning in the work. It refers to an emotional disturbance, linked to the workplace and stress caused by the work environment, with important repercussions, both physical and psychological. It manifests itself preferentially through symptoms of decay and anxiety, causing much of the work casualties.

Burnout syndrome is said to occur most often in the fields of medicine and teaching, in people who have embraced the profession vocationally. As causes, the stress in the workplace is invoked.

And the commentary for the previous section, for the bulling, is applicable to this that neither is new nor is a discovery worthy of being included in the psychiatric nomenclature, which does not contradict the fact that adverse working conditions affect negatively on the personal welfare.

All the sufferings that are expressed through psychic signs have their root in the particular form of the development of the individual, being the unfavourable working conditions just a trigger. In any case, it does seem obvious that a pleasant working environment can be a corrective experience for the person who is inclined to suffer this type of response, although it must be agreed that the bases would already be established and the undesirable circumstances of the work just complete the picture.

Moreover, it is exceptional that the person has not encountered inept leaders throughout his professional career. It would not be wrong for employers to require specific training as a prerequisite to running a business organization. But things are what they are and society, as always, is on the way to perfection, in this field as in the rest.

The shameful examples offered by the public figures, immersed in financial scandals, pursuing without modesty the power as a personal addition and not as a means to translate some ideas for the perfection of the society to which they would have as mission to serve. This behaviour brings as a consequence its discredit and the disenchantment of the administered. Particularly our political class behaves, on these days, like schoolchildren at the recess: forming gangs to confront others. In their public appearances they boast of being ahead, in the polls, as if this were the end of their tasks. Never, but never, even by mistake, slip a worry about the magnificent task they could have at his hands: the citizens' welfare. If these characters are called to be examples, better that God find us confessed.

This confusion also occurs in many unfortunate entrepreneurs to whom life has not allowed to know that, in fact, the companies are like the children: beings in growth that will give in return much more than the sleeplessness that their care has required. And so they live in the disorientation of pursuing a fictitious relevance.

There are those who believe in seeing in the conditions of the vocation a motive for each election. Thus, jocularly, it is said, about the medical vocation, that people who carry an unconscious trait of sadism opt for the surgical specialties; that those who have a tendency towards the sexual curiosity would end up in the gynecological specialty; the specialties of Psychiatry and Psychology would be reserved for those who seek to "heal" themselves, and so on. Finally, all those with an uncontrollable passion for power, you know what path they would take, even if you doubt it, I will tell you that yet as teenagers they would join the youth of a political party.

## d) Asperser's syndrome

In reviewing my school life, I believe that I have always had knowledge that there were students with open dislike for any of the subjects, but never this animosity deserved the establishment of a particular picture in the psychiatric classification.

It seems that we are going back to the descriptive epoch of Psychiatry. Thus, the current manuals describe the so-called Asperger's syndrome of which I have the impression of being an unnecessary psychiatric creation. It simply reflects the fact that a child does not like a particular subject -as he would not want to go to school either- and to refer to these behaviours, apart from being considered problems of the teaching itself and fundamentally the competence of the teachers, I do not see the need to create a new entity. Psychiatry picks up the commentary of a child that he does not like mathematics, for example, and from there it creates a new syndrome: that of Asperger. And issue solved.

Here is an expressive example of the transaction between the aversion produced in the child by the parents' insistence and their passive opposition, all of which is dramatized in the scenario of antipathy towards a certain subject matter.

## e) Allergies

Comparing the medical studies of my time with the present ones, I find very few points of similarity. By then, they were described a series of manifestations, incipient in those days, that are constantly gaining ground in an extraordinary way. I am referring to allergies, which are basically unexpected answers to substances whose contact is familiar to the body but which, on occasions, lead to misguided and diverse responses, such as asthma, conjunctivitis, eczema, etc. As I say, the variety of its presentation is such that a new modality appears daily without its aetiology being known although, as usual, its explanation invokes the genetic reasons, always waiting to be demonstrated.

In my opinion, all types of allergies can be included in the chapter of psychosomatic diseases because the psychological component seems to be determinant.

Allergy to milk or to some of its components, such as lactose, is an eloquent example of the existence of an unconscious rejection of the mother since the milk is the intermediary in the first contact with her and whit the life. It may be objected that psychoanalytic orientation always leads to the same fate: parents, childhood, and the past. It will also be thought that, for such a variety of presentations, the explanations are scarce, but it must be borne in mind that it is not in this section that these simplifications are only given, since the possibilities of expression of any ailment are equally scarce. The immediate response to any type of infection is unspecific, always the same, the increase in the number of leukocytes.

The number of intolerances increases for days. Among them is intolerance to pollen, gluten or celiac disease, lactose and an endless list of them.

## f) Anorexia and Bulimia

This section is one in which you can more clearly observe the clumsiness of the proceeding of Psychiatry. The technique is simple: if a person exhibits a conflict with food and their weight experiences ostensible variations, the therapeutics is immediate: if the problem is reduced to weight loss, force to the seditious to ingest food and prevent voluntary vomiting; if, on the other hand, the result of the insurrection is the increase of weight, keep to himself away from any possibility of satisfying his voracious appetite; as simple as the mechanism of a rattle. Very elemental, is not it?

To the question of why a person may be the subject of this problem, the answer is equally immediate: because it has a perverse attitude. And with these premises begin the calvaries, the prohibitions, the punishments, the weight controls and the isolates in the psychiatric units. And since science presumes that behind each picture there is no psychological conflict - that this is something of psychoanalysts- but a certain ignorance to feed properly, the remedy will be the preparation of experts to teach them: the nutritionists. And as long as things are as they are, it will be well to prohibit the participation of these people in fashion shows so that they do not become vehicles of contagion.

Unfortunately, the dynamics of these states, of easy understanding, are not as elemental as the psychiatric care shows. If there is a matter that, apart from its genuine purpose of nutrition, lends itself to represent something more transcendent, this is the food. If we follow the thread of this reflection we find that the beginnings of life coincide in the same pattern: the child stuck to the mother's breast. Could it be, then, that these striking variations in body weight were the expression of unconscious conflicts in relation to the mother?

## g) Orthorexia

It is a term of new coinage that shelters situations characterized by the obsession to take exclusively foods considered healthy; an obsession that can lead to malnutrition. The person who carries this obsession avoids a series of foods, such as fats, dyes and preservatives.

Dynamically, nothing is different from the tables described above.

## h) Vigorexia

This section in no essential aspect differs from the previous ones. He is also described as an obsession about physical fitness. The problem here, as in the previous ones, is the lack of acceptance of one's own body image. These people react with frantic physical activity, making their life a continuous training, combined with the intake of anabolic in order to boost muscle mass.

In the same way as the solitude which, in its psychological sense, does not refer to the absence of companionship but to the lack of understanding between the psychic instances within the person, in all these pictures, in which there seems to be a repudiation of the body image, what really happens is a disagreement with the way of being in the world, with the estrangement from the goal of being oneself; a conflict that has been displaced towards the body sphere.

## i) Aids

It will be that the passage of the years is responsible for the strangeness that causes me the present. I feel like this with the so-called Immunodeficiency Syndrome. In the early days of my medical studies it seemed everything to be clear: there was a set of diseases with their well-established aetiology, prognosis, and treatment. I could hardly think then that with the passage of time new ones would appear, as it happened in the 80's, with the birth of a curious disease, of uncertain origin, that soon was related to the sexual activity and the consumption of drugs.

It is said to be caused by the human immunodeficiency virus, of African origin. This disease soon aroused strong controversy due to the preponderant role of sex in its origin and propagation. All these factors together, with the prohibition of the use of condoms on the part of the ecclesiastical authority, impressed a religious hue to this disease. It was also called AIDS because of the existence of pink spots and from the beginning it was considered a punishment of God because of depravity, as in Sodom and Gomorrah.

## j) Ebola

In my studies in Microbiology, the professor, an exaggerated and not quite well-intentioned character, summoned us around a fellow who looked through the microscope and with exaggerated signs of being scandalized, shouted, while ridiculing the poor student, "look. Look, at your companion, he is seeing a virus!" Was then when I learned that viruses were only visible through the electron microscope, which was then yet to come. Its diffusion is the one that allows the discovery of new viruses, like the Ebola, responsible for a recent commotion that, like the summer storm, seems to have passed.

Also, the called the Zika virus, which is transmitted by the mosquito and that produces microcephaly, has caused a temporary stir.

## k) The "Restlessness"

If my vanity would remain with sufficient vigour and I preserve, yet, some yearning for protagonism, would borrow from a dear colleague the occurrence of baptizing a quite widespread behaviour, probably more frequent among women, characterized by an uncontrollable activity that does not find rest, with the denomination of the syndrome of "restlessness". It is the attitude of beings in a continuous "without living", in a permanent sigh, in whom the agitation, rather than conducting to a profitable activity, hardly achieves effective goals. They are people to whom life prevents from living in tranquillity but continuously doing things, without being able to sit, calmly, on the couch, doing nothing or scratching their belly on the beach under the sun. It seems that they live to convince to their neighbours that they are effective and that they are not idle.

Going from place to place, without ever finding the destination, seems to be the condemnation that underlies in his ardent eagerness. People for whom the expressions "I have to do" or "I must do" seems to constitute the slogans etched in their minds. With that incessant activity, blames, indirectly, the people of their environment.

If we had to classify such behaviour in the classical style, we would speak of agitated, cyclic or bipolar people. But, since our task is the one of the understanding, we will see in them the maintenance of the everlasting struggle between the instances of the ego and the moral conscience. In the absence of any obligation, they are unable to rest, to enjoy the stillness. The delight of contemplation and leisure is forbidden to them; they are condemned to permanent movement, which Balthasar Gracián has judged, so little charitably, as the passion of fools.

We come from a culture in which leisure is the mother of all vices and in which we should not leave for tomorrow what could be done today.

## 7. DROGADICTION

Like all events in life, the subject of drug addiction also evolves with ups and downs. In the beginning of my training, the consumption of cannabis, familiarly known as marijuana, was a novelty that in a few years grew, spreading to other substances such as heroin, cocaine, amphetamines and other synthetic preparations. Such was the degree of social innocence at that time that, for students on the eve of examinations, and for truck drivers to combat the dream of night travel, we had within our reach an amphetamine, "the Centramine", without it waking some social alarm.

But, as I say, what began with the character of snobbishness soon spread like the plague and, suddenly, the Psychiatry had to find accommodation to these pictures, generally characterized by rebellion and to which few professionals felt some kind of sympathy, because his attention shocks with uncomfortable obstacles, such as the absence of voluntariness, the frequent connection with the world of delinquency and, above all, the lack of understanding of how many professionals were in charge of his attention, accustomed, as they were, to acting inflexibly in the eradication of symptoms. Keep in mind that this type of care is exceptionally presided by the pact and, therefore, the attention against the will is almost a perversion.

A comment before continuing. Pharmacology deals with the effects of the application of various substances on living organisms; Psychology, on the other hand, deals with the dialogue that is established between the substance and the receiving organisms. The data obtained in pharmacology hardly take into account the particularities of the recipient; On the contrary, Psychology deals with the nature of the dialogue established in such a way that it can be observed how the same substance produces disparate effects on different people. In this sense, life runs in a continuous dialogue of the person with herself and with the world and Psychology deals with this dialogue without giving excessive consideration to the substance that at every moment enters in the circulatory stream of the recipient. As I say, for Psychology what is important is the state of the recipient and to his study dedicates the efforts. Life is a journey full of difficulties for which crossing is necessary to have the necessary supports. Well, in this context we must admit that the support will be subject to the state of the person in such a way that we can well consider that, for this tiring journey, any help could be considered as a drug. In some cases it will be the work, in others reading, in others tobacco, in others alcohol, in others the consumption of narcotic substances, in others cosmetics and so on to infinity.

For all these considerations, Psychology can't regard the drug dependence as an exceptional situation. Another quite different matter is the social consideration that deserves the nature of the different supports used in the aforementioned crossing. Work-related addiction does not, at first sight, cause the same harm than cocaine dependence, but this does not mean that there are essential differences in the dynamics of both behaviours.

Not all the phenomena that take place in life are observable by the senses, but, on the contrary, most of them occur beyond their scrutiny. Would we qualify as addicted to the walking stick to a person deprived of mobility in one of his limbs? For what which so logically manifests itself on the physical plane happens also in the psychological one. The greater or lesser strength of a person will be which determines that the kind of supports which have to be used in their pilgrimage through the life, be more or less evolved; that is the only difference. Therefore, it is not possible to approach the subject of the drug, as is usually done, considering the person of the addicted the author of his own addiction.

Drug addiction is another tiring subject. It would seem as if, even in the schoolyard or in the neighbourhood, we continued playing to the game "let's see if you catch me". On the one hand, the police perfects more and more his searching and detecting procedures and, on the other hand, the trafficker's refiners their way of introducing a substance, of scarce original value but that the prohibition elevates it to astronomical amounts. Thus this traffic can, even, to bend laws, to buy governments, to pervert justice and sow corruption wherever it sits.

Considering the number of misadventures that this theme triggers, like the violence of the struggles, the crimes and dramas, it could serve as a hilarious script for a series of comics of the style of "Roberto Alcázar and Pedrín": a derisory succession of comic episodes. But, no, in the press appears daily the news of the "seizure the biggest stash of drug confiscated to date" whose record is constantly being beaten up without that the access to consumption being hampered. And in the shadow of all these "successes" are festering dreadful family dramas, murders, criminal revenge among gangs and the corruption of judges and governments.

If it were not because life was ruled by irrationality, it would be difficult to understand the current scenario of drug dependence. I say this because there should be sufficient experience from the period of the "Dry Law", back in the 1920s, whose implantation brought more horrors than the evils it tried to avoid, until finally it had to be repealed.

In my student years, there in Valladolid, I met a police commissioner, a neighbour of my town. He was a jovial person and, between joke and joke, he told us, to dad and me, the anecdote that a thief had stolen the wallet from the wife of a high dignitary, with the consequent commotion. The commissary assembled the most distinguished pickpockets and indicated them the date and place in which should be deposited. So it was. The authorities know very well that it is more beneficial to exercise some tolerance with smaller offenders than the strict application of the protocol. The police need the confidence of petty thieves, to have under control those of greater rank.

Let us understand, therefore, that all actions, whether socially beneficial or not, have their cause in such a way that the obstruction in the mechanism of substitution of an intolerable world by another fantasized one, must necessarily have its repercussion in the balance of the psychic forces.

What is commented about drugs is valid also for the subject of alcohol, because finally life is a dialogue between objectivity and subjectivity, between desire and prohibition. To whom life has given him sufficient capacity to contain the impulses, he may submit to what is demanded by manners. But this is not always the case since there are circumstances especially unfavourable to the individual, since birth, which make it impossible to submit to the social precepts.

What happened historically with the issue of alcohol can help us to answer the question of whether the legalization of drug use could be the best remedy, I don't say to the underlying conflict in any addiction that belongs to living itself, but the horrors which their consumption causes. Recall us that at the beginning of the last century, and in order to avoid the ills attributed to alcohol consumption, the so-called Dry Law was promulgated and that minutes before it came into force was celebrated by its exalted promoter, the Senator Andrew Volstead, with his unfortunate statement: "Tonight, one minute after twelve, a new nation will be born, a new society in which jails and reformatories will become curiosities of the past". But the reality was very different. Violence broke out, murders multiplied, mafia organizations became powers comparable to institutional ones, and, to top it all, alcohol consumption did not decline. The remedy proved worse than the illness he was trying to cure, so a few years later the law was abolished and life went the way it used to.

This precedent can make us doubt of the effectiveness of the prohibition because, as with cosmetic surgery interventions that cannot stop the passage of time, nor the difficulties of existence. There are no simple solutions to complex problems, and those behind the substance use belong to the formidable difficulties of life. It is not so simple as to be sentenced with conventional phrases like this: “this person has no will" or with the repeated comment that such people "have fallen into the pit of drugs" as if it were a casual accident. Too simple!

## 8. PSYCHOLOGY AND ETHICS

The Ethics, or Normative Philosophy, differs from the Psychology in which the last one studies a phenomenon and that the first judges it. For the purposes of Psychology the ethical propositions cannot interfere at all since their purpose is only to know and in this endeavour nothing can be forbidden to their curiosity. The purpose of knowledge can be so much devoted to know a saint as to an evildoer. Knowing by itself is not, an idle activity, since when the object of knowledge comes to be conscious of the forces that in the penumbra govern the person' life, it experiences the establishment of being unconditional friend with himself.

And this is so because, exposed morality as a series of rules whose follow-up is healthy by itself, we would run into the inconvenience that not everything that could be beneficial is in our hands to do.

On the subject of morality, Freud simplified the problem of good and evil by transferring it to the individual psychological sphere and, within it, to the result of the conflict between the interests of the Ego and the prohibitions against them, including religious doctrines, insecurity of life, obsession and fears of punishment, helplessness, collision of interests between parents and children, uncertainty, etc.

# 9. HEALTH ASSISTANCE

Insisting on the fact that medicine sins of petulance is a reality that I do not think deserves further arguments. Betting for the achievement of the definitive release of the disease, that hopes conquer in the near future thanks to the latest advances in genetic engineering, may be the destiny of the human's hopes. It has not been many years that was deciphered the genetic code, and that the human genome that was completed, a fact from which the most surprising medical advances were expected, but that, for the moment, have not been confirmed. And it is that, perhaps, the existence will persist being this familiar valley of tears.

Advances in genetics have awakened the conquering spirit that every person carries within, making him believe that there will be no limits to his intrepidity and that one day he will be able to be a creator of himself. With the conclusion of the genetic map, it was thought that the last barrier that separated the person from the disease had been demolished. However, it has not been long time since in April of 2003, coinciding with the conclusion of the sequence of the human genome and the explosion of the triumphant enthusiasm that aroused, for that the waters returned to the channel where they used to.

By means of the genetic tests it is aspired to know a series of data such as the diagnosis of diseases and the forecast of its course and prognostic; the anticipation of ailments in healthy people and the foresight of probable hereditary malformations. In the genetic manipulation the hopes of a definitive eradication of the disease are put today. Finally the genetic studies it aspires to eliminate, once and for all, the improperly called mental illnesses, because the academic medicine thinks that they have an organic basis.

The spectacular advances in medical care, preferably in the surgical field, are based on the fantastic development undergone by the physical sciences and the introduction of new materials that lead to the creation of surprising means of exploration and diagnosis. And under the protection of these advances, comes what has always been the dream of medicine: the prevention.

But with the anticipation of the future occurs what has already occurred as soon as man went out into outer space: he assumed that the universe was born at that time, that there was no past and that the thickness of the ozone layer was decreasing and with it, also, the protection to certain harmful radiations, as well as the increase of dermal lesions, like the melanomas. And all this, as it was expected, attributable to the emission of gases from the combustion caused by the improvement of living conditions; again, the recurring conjunction of enjoyment, sin and punishment.

In the uncontrolled consumption of drugs can also be seen a mimicking of the past religious practices because, rationally considered, how to admit that the intake of a substance can offer an explanation about the particular journey of the person from the days of his arrival to this world? It is somewhat comical to think that a clever little pixie, tucked into the bottom of a capsule and working meticulously from the bowels of the organism, could mend the history. Once again, the psychiatric pharmacological prescription reminds us of the parallelism, already mentioned, between this type of practices and religion.

This ingestion of drugs without measure, each for a particular mission, has something of a grotesque. As if each of them were piloted by a sagacious genius, able to go to the precise place and disperse his miraculous principle there. Thus, one tablet for the thyroid, another for circulation, another for sight, another for dizziness, another for bones... All a rosary of tasks, as if the organism were a puzzle and it had to be attended to each piece separately from the others. In addition, it is the fact that the storage of products in households is a high cost of stocks for public finances. The organism is just a unit, it does not works in parts and, in my opinion, that unity is governed by emotions and these, in turn, by biographical references.

Like all that has to do with the anticipation of the future, prevention is a tricky matter. Asked that he was a shepherd who, because of passing a lot of time in the field, he was credited of being an expert meteorological forecaster, about whether it would rain that afternoon, he answered impassively, after look at the sky, that the next day he would give the answer.

I was studying fourth grade when, on the occasion of the subject of Gynecology, I stumbled upon something hopeful that inaugurated a new era in which it would not be necessary to wait for a disease to appear crystallized, completely established. It was the early diagnosis of carcinoma of the cervix by means of the anatomopathological study of the exudation. It is true that vaccines had already brought spectacular advances, although they were confined to infectious disease.

It is possible that, as a result of these findings, the path of prevention, that invades all areas of medical work and floods the advertising space of our television, begins today. For this company, the procedure followed is full of ingenuity; It suffices to note that the passage of the years, deteriorating the body as a whole, the joints cannot be an exception in losing his freshness and be source of discomfort. And once deduced that the cartilage has lost vitality, the remedy is immediate: it will be enough to take preparations of cartilage or its precursors, in the candid belief that is produced what is eaten, and that the digestive laboratory, in charge of metabolizing food and extract their beneficial principles, are at the service of consumer desires. From this simple syllogism will be harmed the sharks without no benefit, in return.

# 10. THE ABORTION

If it were not that the incoherence was an inseparable part of existence, we would be surprised by the fact that at a moment of exaltation of democratic values, such as the present, is denied to the main protagonist, the woman, some kind of management in the so delicate theme of the abortion.

Before approaching this theme, which awakes such lively passions, one must be aware that words have a particular meaning and cannot be slid out of it, because otherwise their use is either a simple error or has the Intentionality to achieve fraudulent purposes. Such is the case of the use of the term murder to refer to abortion, which, by definition, refers to the interruption of a process that leads to birth. It is well noted here that the use of the word murder has the intention of eliminating any other point of view. But above all, the issue of abortion, once exposed to political debate, is left perverted.

Subjected to a purely rational scrutiny, the banner wielded by certain associations contrary to his practice that, without flushing, claim to be in favor of life, has no coherence, because for this statement to make any sense would have to face others that were openly In favour of death. It happens here as in politics where the custom has given by good the qualification of progressive to any orientation of left, with which automatically to the opposite positions are certified like of reactionary.

It does not seem judicious that Psychiatry should intervene in the controversial subject of abortion unless of invading the moral side. For the medicine, the surgical procedure of abortion is today a simple intervention, although this was not always the case, and the history is full of tears, violence and death, when clandestine practice was in the hands of healers.

And when it is affirmed to be in favour of life, what life are we referring to? Because existence, understood as the transit of the person throughout the days between birth and death, is diverse for each being in such way that, encompassed by the same expression, could well lead to confusion. For the being that appears accidentally in the world, the life does not appear to be the same as for who is expected with joy. In both cases there is a life but you can well suspect that their future will not be the same.

In any case, the embryo will remain in the woman's womb for months and it can be thought that, subject to an event that will mediate her life, she should be, before anyone, protagonist. If we speak of freedom, the decision to interrupt the pregnancy is something that is primarily the responsibility of the mother, even if it is an event that, secondarily, affects her partner and to society as a whole.

Able that there is a part of the population that welcomes its avoidance. In addition, the arrival of children not always is the result of voluntary decision of parents. Likewise, nothing is known about the suffering of the unborn. To the children who die at birth the Catholic Church sent them to limbo, not many years ago. From time to time the newscasts give account of parents who immolate their creatures, guided by the intention to avoid their suffering.

Of all the arguments put forward against the interruption of the pregnancy, the most ruthless, the ones who has least regard for the new being, are the ones wielded by those who mourn their loss because "they could have become to be an Einstein or an Anna Pavlova".

In any case, psychiatry has no special authority to intervene in such a controversial subject, which passionate opinions arouse because, with respect to them, as of all those who promote the great debates, its task is fulfilled with individual attention, regardless of The moral qualification that the decisions could deserve. The Psychologist, as much as the others, can have a particular opinion on the various current issues, but he can not rest in the possession of any superior authority or that the options he defends had a greater value, which would constitute the widespread vice of the confusion of the limits of representation. It is the same as in the radio or television gatherings in which some intervener arrogates greater right in the support of his opinion by the fact of having "reflected extensively" on the subject to debate.

Being that with so much emphasis we defend the freedom, it is paradoxical that we show intolerant with those who are in disagreement with the secular customs. We are proud extolling the values of freedom and democracy, and yet how easily we judge the life of our neighbours without knowing their circumstances..! From my adolescence I have the memory of the dramatic episode in which a poor woman died because a clandestine interruption of pregnancy. By then, I thought about the tremendous circumstances that the unhappy woman must have undergone who, without having married, had become pregnant and that, like a leper, was expelled to the street for being the shame of her family.

Considering that the Psychiatry as the discipline that tries to understand behaviours rather than speculate about the freedom to choose one over the other, it is up to the social order to authorize or reject abortion. Psychiatry deals with the understanding the effects of undesirable conditions derived from the obligation of continuing the pregnancy, in the same way that it has to understand the consequences of its interruption without having to opt for any trial. It must be away from the decision, just has to understand.

# 11. THE SUICIDE

Within that passion that governs the people to adjective the behaviour of the neighbour, the suicide has been judged with the most inopportune adjective, the one of cowardice, obviating thus, with a single sentence, the mention to the movers that push to such a dramatic action. The courage, like the cowardice, are, moreover, punctual expressions referred to a certain facts propitiated by historical conditionings but that are present, at least outlined, in every person.

The much-vaunted freedom, which we know does not have its correlate in Psychology, refuses to be applied to these acts to the point that not many years ago the author was buried in spaces outside from the hope to participate in the benefits of eternal salvation.

## 12. EUTHANASIA

The serenity that some people seem to enjoy in the, euphemistically called "third age" is due to the favourable conditions of yesterday, that the expectations of the future are almost null, since the most feared upheavals of life have been left behind. In their heart, they know that practically everything is finished. With the decadence of the instinctual drive all the fears that have accompanied their lives, diminished by the passage of time, have practically disappeared. And, despite of this calm, there are people who prefer to put an end to their existence, a desire difficult to attainable due to the obstacles of an incongruous society that, boasting of a fictitious freedom, is scandalized when it comes to acting accordingly.

Those who have the opportunity to work in homes for the elderly will meet people who, openly and with full consciousness, manifest the desire to end their representation and, disregarding their desires, society insists in trying to maintain their faculties, physical and intellectuals, with the imposition of grotesque exercises that does not even allow them to be at peace with their thoughts and memories.

Fortunately there are a movement, in principle more benevolent, that advocates the right to a dignified death. The realization of this desire, which seems so logical, encounters incomprehensible obstacles, most often belonging to the religious tradition. Counted are the countries -Australia at this time, Holland, the state of Oregon in North America- that have dared to tear down these barriers and have voted a law regulating what is coming to know for a dignified death, authorizing the prescription of lethal preparations to the persons who, in their terminal phase, request it.

However, why should a death be described as "dignified"? Is there an unworthy way to die? Of course there is and takes place daily in hospitals where the endless succession of tests, often without clear guidance or any objective, make the last few dates a painful torture. And it is that, at this point, the medical arrogance behaves with the same despotism with which the religious shepherds once did with their flock, which again falls into a contradiction: on the one hand we are fervent supporters of democracy, of freedom and tolerance and of another we fiercely oppose to a person making the decision to put an end to his own life.

The pretext that causes the person be no the owner to put a date at the end of his life -whose beginning he could not decide, either- is based on the poor argument that the legal practice of euthanasia could lead to abuse.

But let us ask ourselves what measure, what innovation or what modification of the law, could not even bring some excess. But, if we speak of freedom, it seems reasonable that the person be allowed to arbitrate about the end.

# 13. PSYCHOLOGY AND LAW

The boldness to write on this subject is motivated by the desire to present a vision from the field of Psychology, given the frequency with which the legal field seeks its assistance. And as in the field of Psychology, it is pertinent to question the existence of freedom, and the establishment of moral judgments, as also it would be an incoherence to speak of responsibilities, it must be presumed well that all legislation is an artificial elaboration with which Is intended to protect certain assets, such as life, property and coexistence.

The Psychology is in charge of searching for the immediate causes -since the remote ones will always be hidden from our research- from the phenomena under examination; To the Justice to judge whether they can be included in a section of the penal code and, if so, proceed to process and subsequent sentence. Cause is a psychological term; responsibility and fault belong to the administration of justice.

Laws are artificial creations, as well as their application in judicial processes. Judgments are accepted as a form of regulation of coexistence, but this does not mean that we believe faithfully in their truth and that we don't have always the consideration that anyone, under the same conditions as the defendant, would occupy its place. It must be recognized that the work of the judges resembles the leap into the void. Judging is such an annoying matter, with so much difficulty, that the Indian proverb says: "Before judging a person, walks three moons within his moccasins". For all this, the exercise of justice must be carried without real conviction, with the same air of provisionality that characterizes the existence.

In the whirlwind of daily life, people are prompted to track down the behaviours in search of explanation to hypothetical errors without falling into the account of the futility of such an endeavour, since again it falls into the trap of the assumption of the existence of free will. This eagerness is particularly accentuated in the essays on history.

Legislative work aspires to be of such a nature that any criminal act should be so precisely fixed in the code, so mathematically enshrined in legislation that all judges, irrespective of their personalities, arrive at identical sentences in the same event. But since this does not happen and the sentences vary depending on the judges who dictate them, it is necessary to emphasize the importance of their personality.

In any case and given the impossibility of scrutinizing the personality of the magistrate with total reliability, it is possible to point out blunders of the great calibre as the one that ends a sentence for drug possession: "the accused will be placed In freedom but is condemned to receive psychiatric therapy" or the opinion that dared to include in the verdict that says: "The rape is less crime when the raped is not a virgin". There are also judges who, disoriented about the limits of their representation, come to interpret even the hidden desires of the accused.

The judge is, finally, another official, with its particularities but with no special prerogative or distinction. Everyone, as children, still play to the professions and shops games. Also the judge plays to impart justice and although their opinions have a significant impact on people's lives, the same argument could be made in the case of the doctor, the fireman, the policeman, the pilot, etc. Neither the judge can be considered an exception because of the position that represents, to express the complaint that a high magistrate said: "For a magistrate it can be insulting to travel in tourist class".

There are in our society a series of inadmissible facts that have nothing to do with the administration of justice and yes with the childish games of school recess. I am referring to the irrational creation of groups, such as the associations of "Judges for Democracy" or the "Association of Judges Francisco de Vitoria" as if they both had a task other than to ensure the proper functioning of justice. Following this disorganized way of working, we could speak of the medical for the health group, pilots against air catastrophes, firefighters against the fire, plumbers against the rupture of pipelines, architects against the collapse of buildings. A delirious exercise of stupidity, although in this sense they would only continue the course of the political class whose aim is to defeat the opposing party, not to contribute to the general welfare.

Psychological assessment, accepting the inability to gag a person in a name, can only be understood in terms of need. The judge "needs" reports that, in essence, are only a way of sharing responsibility. If it is accepted that the person is unclassifiable, the psychiatric reports have a misleading validity.

The psychologist receives the person who comes to the consultation, listens to his story and makes an explanation but, in my opinion, it is not within his job to point out that someone is "not well" or that "is in need of treatment ...". This way, apart from invading other limits, is tortuous because, even in the case of having the assent of the other person, the consultations would be lost in the impossible demonstration of what is "being well or bad".

Many lines back, we leave the pair of crazy lovers in their reverie. A recess, that nature grants in order to shore up their eagerness, which is the continuity of the species. But already, with the established roles, life puts an end to that temporary permit to claim them to its company. Then the "with you bread and onion" vanishes to occupy the forefront of the enterprise the conjunction of interests, always looking at the propagation and permanence of the human race. Thus, the formation of the couple follows a shared pattern. Each of the components, coming from different worlds, will have to suffer the difficulties inherent in the company of joining the divergent forces towards a common destiny: the raising of children. Only this can be the reason that two people from different backgrounds can integrate their energies.

This adjustment company always starts with identical nostalgia and protests: "the food is not the same as the one made by mom" or "you do not love me as before". And so, with these small protests begins to weave the plot of the continuity of the species, with the expensive and delicate threads of a new alliance.

The destiny of the pair transcends the particular views of each of its components and, since everything is really destined for the permanence of the species, soon the children appear. And in relation to them parents usually behave, in the worst cases, as if they were a belonging and so it is observed how often the parents put on their children their failed hopes, causing comparisons and creating, in this way, the disagreement and the rivalry, in clear disregard for the poet's warning: "children come from you but they are not yours"

The commentary on the following quotation is, by no means, moralizing since we have agreed to leave all judgment aside, It's not a critic either; It Is simply testimony to the degree of severity that life can reach. Well, a prestigious figure of psychiatric discipline declared in a newspaper that his children interested him while they were discovering the world, but from the age of six they became a nuisance. And next he added that he felt more affected by not having obtained the chair than by the circumstance of his son's death.

It is said that Hegel had the opinion that children are never aware of the efforts of the parents and his debt for to them. Again this quotation removes us from the purpose of the understanding to move us to the sphere of judgments. Understanding has nothing to do with debts or gratitude, although admitting the need for relief, the philosopher's own argument could be used in the opposite sense, because the children would be indebted to parents if life were a good and they had come voluntarily; otherwise, the children would be the creditors. The causes precede the effects.

Within the family the role of the mother is essential. She is the one who receives the new being and in the expression of his face, en the way of her being, is configured his future. If her face shows fascination, the journey of the newcomer will run in peace, even with the natural difficulties of life. Her handling, kissing and caressing will be, for the infant, a safe protection against many future anxieties, safeguarding of undesirable dermatological manifestations and immunity against asthma, among many other bodily evils.

It is known that Kant was accompanied by an extraordinary concern for health. Perhaps the premature death of his mother was latent in his methodical behaviour and meticulous ordering of his habits.

Allusions to the figure of the mother are endless. Thus, Calderón in his work, "La Vida es Sueño", puts on the lips of his character: "I dreamed that in another, more flattering state I saw myself," in clear allusion to the mother. Between sobs, she introduces us to life, and if her being in it allows her, she will dissipate the initial disconcert of the infant and the uneasiness that the strangeness of life provokes. And at night, when the separation is allied with the darkness, the newcomer will not hesitate to run to the bed where she is, and in the bay of her arms will be diluted his most violent nightmares. She is the first face we perceive and the one that will remain forever in our retinas.

The rest of the days of life will pass in the same way as the walking of the donkey chasing the carrot or behind a vicarious objective, like love, studies or profession. Only at the end we`ll realize that the journey has been a prolonged persecution of the returning to the lost paradise.

The woman seems to address the man although it is only a momentary detour because she has also the tendency to come back, to return to the place that never should have been abandoned. Man, on the other hand, "chooses" a substitute of the mother but, also, waiting for the definitive return to her. The mother is, in short, the unique opportunity to experience the unconditional love; Outside of her will be possible its pursuit, but not its achievement. This idea lends the extraordinary fascination to songs, like the Irish Danny Boy or the sublime Solveig's song?

This excellent figure is present in poetic compositions, in the song's lyrics and in all artistic creations. Even in politics, because how to explain the bloodthirsty behaviours in claim of a land, of language and the religion?

The daughter's love for the mother has a submissive component because, secondarily, she goes to the father and then goes in search of the male. The love of the son by the mother is the precursor of the model that will continue with the wife.

It is unlikely that any person has ever suffered from jealousy throughout their existence because, however fortunate your experience may have been, at some point the hopes had to be been defrauded. Moreover, since jealousy is the consequence of the need to be loved, no matter how favourably the different stages of development have gone through, the experience of painful separation has had to be inevitable. Inescapable dependence carries with it the fear of losing anchorage. Therefore, one could only understand the ignorance of jealousy in who has never depended and could boast of not needing to be loved, which is a chimerical circumstance.

The jealousy, common reason for psychological consultation, is usually settled with reasoned considerations and some drug, since they are barely understood despite its overwhelming simplicity. Thus, the client leaves the consultation affirmed in the idea that being jealous is part of his person, as it were an inseparable characteristic of his nature. However, the careful listening of his story shows us, first of all, to a person who pretends the impossible: that his partner ceases to exist to turn around him, like a satellite or, what is the same that would cease to be a person. And when the partner of the jealous person agrees to such request, only possible in very tight spaces of time, checks that not even so the torments are appeased; he, or she, will always find a detail that will confirm infidelity.

Let us now compare this behaviour with that which takes place in the couple that evolves towards the constitution of a true friendship enterprise in which each one is satisfied that the other has its own life, that no one loses any trait of its personality. Thus, the couple will constitute the company formed by two loyal partners.

Why, then, is it so difficult to access this state that would be the most desired? Simply because the journey of people's lives is not guided by reason, so we can ask what irrational elements may be responsible for such disorientation? Coming to this point, let's hold of some literary source. Thus, the comment, attributed to Jacinto Benavente, who says: "the jealous, never is by what he sees; with what is imagined is enough".

From this quote one can deduce the hypothesis that jealousy could be independent of the behaviour of the person whom one believes to love. And if this were a correct deduction, we would have to admit that the jealousy could be prior to the knowledge of the couple and that the actual person is only the screen on which they are projected. Well, if the jealousy were prior to the knowledge of the person who is believed to be its origin and that the experience of them has already been lived in another setting and in another time, we can only ask when and with whom the experience took place originally.

Jealousy does not start from the fear of not being corresponded since this is one of the vicissitudes of life;

On the contrary, the jealousy is prior to deception. The jealous -we all are or have been in a greater or lesser extent- starts from the certainty that he will be betrayed. It is like the anticipation of what will inevitably happen and is that nothing can be feared of the future that has not already taken place in the past.

But let's go step by step. Let us try to crumble this phenomenon of jealousy. Let us first say that, applying the principle that distinguishes the being from the staying; we must speak of who suffers from this torture as someone who stays jealous, not being jealous. And, why does he suffer from this tribulation? To answer this question let us try to highlight the characteristics of the phenomenon itself. In the first place, the jealous behaves as if had the right that the "beloved" must obligatorily correspond in the desired form, only in this way can it be understood that a person arrogates the power to spy and interfere in the intimacies of the other.

Admitting, therefore, that no legislation grants the right to be loved, nor obligates anyone to love, it is necessary to investigate in some antecedent that would explains such an unreason. And that search leads directly to the stage where all this seems to find a satisfactory explanation. Of course I am referring to the framework in which the first relations with the mother are developed. Indeed, there the adult unreason becomes reasonable. The child has all the "right" to be loved and for him the mother has the "obligation" to love it. Then, jealousy reproduces in adulthood the way it has been "loved" in the early stages of life.

Those who suffer from jealousy consume the time, from morning to night, trying to confirm that their suspicions are founded. But, of course, as the investigations pursue the discovery of the authorship of a crime and it has been committed previously, the fate cannot be other than the dismantling of a relationship of precarious beginnings. Jealousy is nothing more than unexpressed hatreds; hatreds hidden under the layer of a false interest.

Although complementary, another way of approaching the issue of jealousy is one that finds its foundation in considering the couple the referee who dictates who is chosen between two or more candidates, a circumstance that, too, renews the children's rivalries propitiated by the parents' lack of tact. The essence of jealousy is the fact of being tested for to be elected.

But it is also that the argument that the jealous wields is the immense love that he feels for the person who, in his judgment, to such unjust tests submits to him. Such love, however, is a kind of attachment with clear childhood traits, it is a love stopped in the first stages of life, as corresponds to the narcissistic type of love. The jealous person experiences attraction that we could very well qualify as "by delegation", in which the reality of the other person remains outside his knowledge.

## 14. THE FAMILY

Many lines back, we leave the pair of turtledoves in their reverie; a recess that nature grants in order to shore up its eagerness, which is the continuity of the species. Already then, with the well established roles, life puts an end to that temporary permit to claim them for to serve his purposes. Then, the rapture of "all my life is you" vanishes to occupy the foreground the desire to join forces, always looking at supreme interest what is the propagation and permanence of the human race. Thus, the formation of the couple follows a shared pattern. Each of the components, coming from different worlds, will have to experience the difficulties inherent in the enterprise of joining the divergent forces towards a common destiny: the raising of children. Only this could be the reason for that two people coming from different backgrounds want to integrate their energies.

This adjustment always starts with identical nostalgia and protests: "this apple pie is not the same as the one made by mom" or "you do not want me as before." And so, with these small protests begins to weave the plot of the continuity of the species, with these expensive and delicate threads of a new alliance.

The destiny of the couple transcends the particular views of each of its components and, since everything is really destined for the permanence of the species, soon the children appear. And in relation to them, parents often behave, in the worst case, as if they were a belonging and so it is often observed how they place their ill-fated hopes on them, leading to comparisons and creating, in this way, the disagreement and rivalry, in clear disregard for the poet's warning: "children come from you but they are not yours."

The comment of the following quotation, in no way has a moralizing eagerness since we have agreed to abandon all judgment, not even wants to be critical; is simply a testimony to the degree of severity that life can achieve. Well, a prestigious figure of the psychiatric discipline told, in a newspaper's interview, that his children interested him as they were discovering the world, but from the age of six they became a nuisance. And next he added that he felt more affected by not having obtained the chair than by the circumstance of the son's death.

It is said that Hegel commented that the children are never aware of the effort of the parents and the debt to them contracted. Again the quotation removes us from the purpose of understanding to move us to the sphere of judgments. Understanding has nothing to do with debts or gratitude, although admitting the need for relief, the philosopher's own argument could be used in the opposite sense, sons would be indebted to the parents if life were a good and if they had come voluntarily; otherwise, the children would be the creditors. The causes are always before their effects.

Within the family, the role of the mother is essential. She is the one who receives the new being and in the expression of her face, in her way of being, is configured his future. If her face shows fascination, the journey of the newcomer will run peacefully, even with the natural setbacks of life. Her handling, her kisses and caresses will be for the infant the best protection against many future anxieties, the safeguarding of undesirable dermatological manifestations and the immunity against asthma, among many other bodily evils.

At this respect, It is well known the fact that Kant was accompanied all the life by an extraordinary concern for his health. Perhaps the premature death of the mother was latent in his methodical behaviour and the meticulous ordering of his habits.

The allusions to the figure of the mother are endless. Thus, Calderon de La Barca, in his work "Life is Dream", puts on the lips of one character: "I dreamed that in another more flattering state I saw myself", in a clear allusion to the mother, because, between sobs, she introduces us to life and, if her way of being allows her, will dissipate the initial disconcert of the infant and the uneasiness that causes his opening to the life. And at night, when the separation is allied with the darkness, the newcomer will not hesitate to run to the mother's, and in the dock of her arms will dilute his most violent nightmares. She is the first face we perceive and the one that will remain forever in our retinas.

The rest of the days of life will pass in the same way as the donkey that goes behind the carrot, after a substitutive compensation, like love, studies or professions. Only at the end, we will realize that the tour really has been an incessant persecution for the return to the lost paradise.

Subsequently, in the course of development the woman seems to address the man, although it is only a momentary detour because in it, too, the tendency to return, to go back to the place that never had to be abandoned, rules. Man, on the contrary, "chooses" a substitute for the mother, but also, waiting for the definitive return to her. The mother is, in short, the unique opportunity to experience unconditional love; out of her will be possible their pursuit, but not their achievement. This idea lends the extraordinary fascination to some poignant songs, such as the Irish Danny Boy or the sublime Solveig's song?

The mother's figure is almost omnipresent in the poetic compositions, in the lyrics of innumerable songs and in the majority of the artistic creations. Even in politics, because how else to explain the bloodthirsty behaviours in claim of a land, a language and a religion?

The daughter's love for the mother has a submissive component because, secondarily, she goes towards the father for, then, to go searching for the man. The love of the child for the mother is the precursor of the model that will continue in the couple.

Being the mother so needed, It is unlikely to find a person that has ever suffered from jealousy throughout their existence because, for much fortunate that had been their experience, at any point their hopes had to be snubbed. Moreover, since jealousy is the consequence of the need to be loved, no matter how favourably the different stages of development have gone through, because the experience of painful separation has had to be inevitable. The Inescapable dependence carries with it the fear of losing the anchorage. Therefore, it could only be understood the ignorance of the jealousy in those that never had to be dependent and could boast of not need at all of to be loved; a chimerical circumstance.

In the psychiatric consultation, jealousy is usually attended by reasoned considerations and the prescription of drugs, since they are barely understood despite their overwhelming simplicity. Thus, the client leaves the query entrenched in the idea that being jealous is part of his person as an inseparable characteristic of his nature, such as having a stain on his skin or dark haired. However, the careful listening of his story shows, first of all, someone who pretends the impossible: that his partner ceases to exist as a person to turn around him, like a satellite; to stop being a person. And when the partner of the jealous person agrees to such an impossible request, only feasible in very tight spaces of time, he proves that even the torments are not appeased; he, or she, will always find a detail that will confirm the infidelity.

Let us now compare this behaviour with that which takes place in the couple that evolves towards the constitution of a true friendship in which each one is just satisfied that the other has his own life, that he has not lost any trait of his personality. Thus, the couple will be formed by two loyal partners.

Why, then, is it so difficult to access this state that would be the most desired? Simply because the journey of people's lives is not guided by reason, so we can ask what irrational elements may be responsible for such disorientation. At this point, let us appeal to some literary source. Thus, the comment, attributed to Jacinto Benavente, who says: "the jealous, never is by what he sees; is enough with what he imagines"

From this quote one can establish the hypothesis that jealousy could be independent of the behaviour of the person of whom one believes to be in love. And if this were a correct deduction, we would have to admit that the jealousy could be prior to the knowledge of the couple and that the person to whom they were addressed is only the screen on which they were projected. Then, if the jealous were prior to the knowledge of the person who the jealous believes to have originate them and that the experience of them has already been lived in another setting and in another time, we can only ask when and with whom took place the first experience.

Jealousy does not start from the fear of not being reciprocated since this is one of the unavoidable vicissitudes of life; on the contrary, jealousy is prior to deception and is not triggered, but they are already. The jealous -and we all have suffered then to a greater or lesser extent- start from the certainty that one will be betrayed. It is like the anticipation of what will inevitably happen. But nothing can be feared of the future that has not already taken place in the past.

But let's go step by step. Let us try to analyze this phenomenon of jealousy. But before this, let us say that, applying the principle that distinguishes staying from being, we must speak of who suffers from this torture as someone who stays jealous, but not is jealous. And why does he suffer from this tribulation? To answer this question let us try to highlight the characteristics of the phenomenon itself. In the first place, whoever that suffers from jealousy behaves as having all rights over the "beloved" in such a way that he had the obligation to accept his wishes as if he were a slave. Only thus can it be understood that a person arrogates to himself the power to spy and to interfere in the intimacies of the other. Admitting, therefore, that no legislation grants the right to be loved, nor obligates anyone to want, it is necessary to investigate in some antecedent that explains such an unreason. And that search leads directly to the stage where all this seems to find a satisfactory explanation. Of course I am referring to the framework in which the first relations with the mother are developed. Indeed, there the adult unreason becomes reasonable. The child has all the "right" to be loved and for him the mother has the "obligation" to love him. Then jealousy reproduces in adulthood the way it has been "loved" in the early stages of life.

Those who suffer from jealousy consume time, from morning to night, trying to confirm that their suspicions are well founded. But, of course, as the investigations pursue the discovery of the authorship of a crime and it has been committed previously, fate can not be other than the dismantling of a relationship of precarious beginnings. Jealousy is nothing but hatred not expressed, hatred hidden under the veneer of false interest.

Although complementary, another way of approaching the origin of jealousy is the consideration of the parents as referees who chose between two or more candidates, a circumstance that easily arouses the children's rivalries. The parents' lack of tact propitiates the development of the jealousy. The root of jealousy is in the fact of being compared before being loved.

The argument that the jealous wields is the immense love that he feels for the person to whom such unjust tests he submits. Such kind of love, however, is a kind of attachment with clear infantile features, it is a love stopped in the first moments of life, as corresponds to the narcissistic type of love. The jealous person experiences attraction that we could very well qualify as "by delegation", in which the reality of the other person remains outside his knowledge.

# 15. EPILOGUE: IN THE SUNSET

From the incessant dialogue that the person maintains with himself, with an inside part, starts the initiative of writing this summary of how much has been my professional life and of the conclusions to which I have arrived is evident. The fact that I begin with this introduction, apparently without sense, is because it serves me for two purposes: firstly, to make clear that nothing contained in these lines is critical with other ways of seeing this subject for I am well aware that the vanity and the competitive spirit of my beginnings prevented me from seeing more clearly the meaning of all the stories offered to me. Second, because I don't aspire to achieve any praise or recognition.

This warning is particularly pertinent to the study of Psychology which deals with manifestations of spiritual suffering which are expressed in a complex and apparently changing form, unlike other disciplines, such as descriptive Anatomy, for example, that deals with the study of physical accidents objectives and stable of the body. The first, the Psychology, has to be helped with the analysis, while the second, the Anatomy, is satisfied with the meticulous description of accidents. In the first the subjective factor is unavoidable, in the second practically nonexistent.

Like other disciplines, Psychiatry has its own terminology which, in general, is unkind and simple, and often hurtful and boastful. I can say that my journey through this field has been spent in the purification of this artificial language, discarding the "ornamental" and seeking simplicity, but always guided by the initial intuition that human manifestations should have a logical relation and accordance with the biographical precedents, until to acquire a complete meaning.

This process has been favoured by other factors, such as the passage of time that has been simplifying our way of being with ourselves and, at the same time, the cooling of the ardour that in youth muddies the understanding. With the passing of the years the needs and the zeal of protagonism are relegated to a second plane, freeing the understanding from the passions of existence and contributing, also, that the psychic manifestations appear less distorted. Here happens like in customs between countries in peace and in the process of creating larger units: that there is less vigilance and, therefore, one has no need to camouflage the few prohibited goods.

Thus, the chimera of the success is released of its charms as happened to "Sinuhe", subjugated by the spell of Nefernefer. At last is installed the tranquillity that allows the observation of the facts as they are presented, without the old ornaments once needed.

Throughout these pages I have doubted, on many occasions, between the use of the terms Psychiatry and Psychology. The first, Psychiatry (from the Greek psyche, soul and iatréia, healing) is responsible for the study and treatment of mental illnesses, the second, the Psychology, (from Greek, psycho, soul and logos) in charge to the study of psychic facts.

Due to the disgust that has always produced me the term of mental illness, as it is inappropriate, discriminatory and unfair, I have preferred to speak of Psychology, even taking into account that both disciplines have well-differentiated origins and developments. To obtain the title of psychiatrist is required a previous degree in Medicine, which is not the case for the practice of Psychology. Because of this, the first is closer to the bed of the patient and next to its end, which may confer a particular character that the Psychology, more theoretical, does not have. But the fact that Psychiatry has not come out of its organicist obsession and the use of drugs, leads me to prefer the use of the term Psychology.

Throughout my journey, much of the psychiatric lingo has disappeared from my vocabulary, along with the replacement of the white dressing gown. Also, who comes to the consultation has undergone successive mutations; first he was the sick, then the patient, later the client, to finally stay in what is, a person. It has been a debugging process in which the forms and choice of words has undergone an important filtering.

Because, in my opinion, there are no so-called mental illnesses and the fact that they are mentioned with great profusion is due only to the human limitation, to their haste, to the need to put a label under each phenomenon, as was done with each geographical feature and each variety of plants. Suffering, in the spiritual sense of the term, is not the consequence of any stigma that is not attributable to the fierceness of one's life. It is not true that there are people who, in themselves, carry anomalies that can be put in psychiatric nosology.

The term mental illness is an artificial creation referred to situations in which, for the understanding, there has been a disconnection between effects and their causes, so that in whom this circumstance occurs -in everyone, to a greater or lesser extent- believe to be authors and protagonists of the sufferings that afflict to them. Something similar that happens to the mules of the mine, who, through endless days of darkness, forgot to have seen the bright meadows of their foal days. Thus, the person can come to believe the falsehood that he never knew the light and that blindness is his essence.

Also my journey through the exercise of Psychiatry has strengthened the scepticism and critical spirit that I can recognize already in my early years. Thus, I have always found the assertion derived from the undeniably genial Darwinian observations that natural selection chooses the best endowed to survive, and that because it seemed to me that "in the best endowed", Is highlighted a virtue and not the consequence of random. Consequently, I wondered: what happens, then, to the salmon that, upstream, ascending on the prey, falls into the jaws of the bear? I was undoubtedly struggling in irrational rebellion, attributing merit to what was simply the product of mere description. In the face of chance is not worth reason or merit.

The aforementioned scepticism, which has always accompanied me, will be responsible for seeing in the approach to ambulatories a similarity with the religious pilgrimages of yesteryear. To the dispensaries seem to go the same faithful who used to go to the temples, and with the same purpose: to find the miracle of salvation, now displaced to the field of the health god,

On the other hand, doctors have also been ready to be a replacement for the priests, both for their dogmatism and for their pride. As an inevitable consequence, in view of this scientific-religious atmosphere, the sick-believers are quick to accept the claims of the sage doctors, who refusing to accept that the true advances of medicine come directly from the portentous developments of physics and of chemistry. The Dr. Molina Núñez, founder of "Peña Retama", commented that Psychiatry sins from dogmatism and lacks of philosophy and poetry.

And it is that medicine suffers from simplicity and is not very attentive when assessing physical facts, as is emphasized in recent events, such as the so-called contagion by Ebola and, in general, in all infectious processes in which It neglects the value that the conditions of the host can have in the final result of the aggression.

The future of any invading agent is decided by the result of the two factors at stake: the reaction of the person receiving the external insult and the characteristics of the invading agent. The end result of an infectious process is not the same in the third world societies as in the affluent ones of the West.

When is said that the great Alexander Fleming have saved many lives with the discovery of the Penicillin, a part of reality is rightly highlighted, because too many lives were saved by the progress of living conditions, like the mass production of food, the improvements in working conditions, establishment of holiday periods, progress in the construction of households, reduction of uncertainty through social benefits and the provision of insurance, etc. All these factors are decisive when assessing the increase in life expectancy.

Because, in my opinion, there is a factor, the anguish, that it is not quantifiable, as it happens in the case of body temperature or in the count of red blood cells, cannot be given the attention it deserves. I refer to the level of anguish that should not be confused with what is commonly called stress, which refers more to the burden because of external causes, such as excessive work and poor rest, with which nothing has to do, since the physical effort, as stronger it may be, do not create anguish. For there to be anguish there must be a confrontation between internal instances. Although it is extremely frequent to point out external events as causes of anguish and nothing further from reality. Anguish is the inherent and inseparable ingredient of life.

Incidentally, and since the term stress is so lavishly used, I would like to point out that, apart from the conceptual inaccuracy mentioned in the previous paragraph, there is another, no less transcendent, that concerns to its remedy, because to a wrong approach, the following corrections are equally erroneous.

As stress is related to excessive activity, either by the objective demands of life like the need to attend to two jobs throughout the day, the remedy will be that of the repose. But if what is there is the anxiety, the remedy, that for the stress was adequate, it will be totally counterproductive in the case of anguish.

Against the stress is recommended practices of control, such as those derived from Zen philosophy, yoga, meditation, contemplation and a whole series of exercises, coming mostly from eastern culture. But when there is a picture of anguish, these measures will further accentuate the excessive control that inevitably underlies. The fundamental deference between stress and anguish is that the former has its main engine in external factors and the second translates always the domain of the Superego over the Self.

The new being opens its eyes to the world in the midst of the greatest helplessness. He cannot manage that the hunger is calmed when is needed, that the thirst is punctually satisfied, that the temperature is in agreement with what is required. The uncertainty about the satisfaction of the need, that the new being is unable to control, establishes the birth of anguish.

From there, appears the despair. Because despair is the consequence of waiting, and what else can the infant do but trust that his needs will be satisfied? These urgencies, basic at the beginning -food, cleanliness and warmth-, are associated with the person who comes to his aid, usually the mother, and very soon appears the painful notion of impotence, of separation, and finally the despair and the feeling of anguish. Freud commented on the anguish that a simple graphical way of understanding it was the mental representation of a child lost in a large market.

Being the life of the person a path that runs from the mother's arms to death, it is logical to think that the fear accompanies him, to a greater or lesser extent, throughout his pilgrimage. And that is why the phenomenon of anguish is an inseparable companion in the lives of people and not something that happens to some and not others. The despair, the mortal disease, as is described by Kierkegaard, is the inevitable suffering of the spirit. In this regard, when the psychiatrist attends to a desperate person, he cannot act as he does in organic medicine, particularly in the physical traumas in which the onset of an injury can be established, but keeping in mind that the despair of a person that comes to de consulting room is not new, that he was already desperate.

When in the beginning of my medical studies I thought of the psychiatric specialty as an option, I immediately realized that I had no choice because I was already trapped by the curiosity of the possible explanation underlying all the behaviours. Even in the beginning of my life, my idea was that all behaviours, even the most extravagant ones, should have a simple explanation and, although that faith went through moments of hesitation, as when I attended a psychiatry class in the mental hospital, was finally strengthened in the contact with new forms of approach to the discipline.

We have the propensity to reduce to a single factor the variants of human behaviour. For example, it is said that power moves the world or that it is love which drives the springs of human eagerness and others see in vanity and selfishness the true engines. Fortunately, the passage of time has allowed the creation of a doctrinal body that understands all possible forms of manifestation without the need to resort to no moral judgment.

The nest is the shelter from which the bird appears to life after a long period of incubation and from there begins the journey without a return ticket. An irresistible pressure pushes him into the future; Is part of the same "vis-a-tergo" that drives the blood through the bloodstream. With the breaking of the egg the bird knows for the first time the separation and thus begins the walk of life, starting from the symbiosis with the mother, before experiencing the inclemency of the weather and the need. It is the first tear of life. The future separations will be mere repetitions, and in all of them there will be, in a greater or lesser degree, a hidden desire for return. Within this same scheme will be able to understand all the diverse appearances of the human conducts. The cut of the umbilical cord marks the definitive separation and the exile of the paradise.

Reluctantly the being will be propelled into the future without possibility of return and in that way will arises the need to build the project of being oneself, which is nothing more than the aspiration to be situated sheltered from the exasperating and uncontrollable need.

What has hitherto been written is in no way a reproach to the state of things; Is simply a comment, the exudation of some bad moods that involves the fact of living. I do not doubt about the good faith of mankind: it would be incongruous with the idea expressed in these pages about existence, because the widespread opinion of an existence governed by an almighty and perverse will that governs arbitrarily the fate of people is a folly. Recent events, such as the holocaust of mad cows, the alarm caused by the outbreak of atypical pneumonia, the malignancy of the radiation of mobile telephony and a number of other cases, highlight the defencelessness of the human race and its ancestral subordination to the guilt and to the sin.

For if, through all this writing, I maintain - always within my restricted professional experience - that the protagonism of the person in the existence is no more than an illusion, it would hardly be accommodated with the belief that our present would be better if powerful wills would not have distorted the course of events. No, things are what they are and are as a consequence of the uncontrollable winds of history. The attribution of facts to minds divided between good and bad is a childish simplification. We are, as humanity has always been, in a phase of its evolution, with its particularities.

Coinciding with the weakening of the religious spirit, arrogance has displaced the servitude and humiliation characteristics of the recent past, perhaps for the sake of a more notorious presence of the person in the affairs of life. It is a true revolution that, like all, is provisionally nourished by a great number of excesses, as can be seen in the striking simplicity with which those responsible for human misfortunes are identified.

This arrogance is present in the new ways of expressing the inevitable subjection to the conditions that life decrees. Thus, frequently is heard that such a person is struggling against the cancer, that he has faced it and that even has defeated him. And in all the preceding statements mention is made of a delirious capacity that surely has as purpose the exaltation of the, more than dubious, existence of the will and its uneven distribution among the creatures.

But, before addressing the issue of the existence, or not, of the will, let's make a little introduction. It is known that, topographically, Freud divided the virtual space of the mind into three regions: unconscious, preconscious and conscious. In the first are stored the affections that have not been able to emerge to the field of consciousness and which, repressed, restrict the mental performance, finally causing the symptoms. The region of the preconscious, on the contrary, harbours everything that is not at the immediate disposal of the individual although without having suffered the effects of repression. The third, the conscious space, is where everything that the individual can dispose of at will is lodged.

At the same time, the psychic apparatus was conceived as the framework of interaction of the two main psychic agents: the Ego and the Super-ego, whose functions are well known. The first, the Ego, is referred to the most genuine part of the person who struggles to approach the ideal of being oneself in dispute with the Superego, or moral conscience, which is the depository structure of all vicissitudes during the course of the education process and whose greater or less rigidity is responsible for the internal dialogue, that sustains the person throughout his life, be disturbing or peaceful.

In Western societies, many physical manifestations have practically disappeared because of spectacular advances in living conditions, such as chilblains, tuberculosis, rickets, rheumatic deforming pictures, vitamin deficiency and persistent migraines, among others. In exchange, new ones have flourished, such as the growing variety of allergies.

In the same way to what happened on the physical plane, also in the psychic structures is experiencing a remarkable evolution, fruit of which the pictures that reflect the spiritual suffering appear more diffuse, so little static that barely resist the passage of days in the psychiatric nomenclature.

Descriptions of classical treatises, such as the populations installed in the so-called "rooms of deeps" of psychiatric hospitals, have become volatilized. The same is happening with some classical description such as the various types of Epilepsy, Huntington's chorea, Sydenham's chorea, Parkinson's disease, and Alzheimer's disease, which, if not fully eradicated, are in clear retreat.

The trajectory of this evolution allows us to predict that the area of the unconscious will occupy less "space" in favor of the conscious, so that the symptoms of the spiritual sufferings will approximate to the natural manifestations of the variations of the mood and they can be understood of a natural form without the need for interpretation.

In the same way that the improvement of living conditions has practically eliminated fearsome diseases, such as tuberculosis, syphilis and measles, also in the psychic sphere, the weakening of prohibitions, parallel to the decline in the weight of religions and relaxation of censorship, will make spiritual manifestations less distorted and thus more directly accessible to understanding. Consequently, the phenomenon of anxiety will be less intense. This unstoppable progression will bring with it that the behaviour of people will be more vigorously guided by rational and conscious elements.

His psychiatric symptom will disappear when the protests it transmits are not censored or prevented from manifesting, because the symptom tortuously translates a complaint. This coming age could be christened as of the agony of the symptom.

The abundance of food, hygiene, improvement of working conditions and housing, to a greater extent than the strict medical advances -most of them driven by technological advances- are the drivers of this change. Because, in my opinion, the action of psychiatric drugs can be reduced to the effects of sedation and hypnosis, beyond which nothing else can be expected, except of being new shackles that paralyze, even more, the movements towards the attainment of the purpose of "being oneself". Faith in antidepressants is a mere illusion.

Predictably, the intensity of the symptom of anxiety will be decreasing as society acquires higher levels of security. Always in my opinion, is the anguish the capital symptom from which the others derive, so what we mean by depression, as well as the subsequent psychotic manifestations will experience a drastic decline.

When I started medical studies, to talk about "somatization" -which is the transformation of psychic energy into physical manifestations-, was like, for a religious, to fall into sacrilege, even though the nature offers samples of its existence, like the sadness is the precursor of tears. The passage of the years has been strengthening its recognition and enhancing its importance to the point that there is no somatic disease in which the importance of emotional factors is not highlighted. A course otherwise predictable since, if the person is the fusion of two inseparable substances, spirit and matter, it is natural that the movements of each of them have their resonance on the other.

Many of the diseases considered physical, in which aetiology is still invoked even organic alterations, are the result of emotional cataclysms, which in no way diminishes its malignity. Thus, I am convinced that cancer, sclerosis, degenerative diseases, allergies and asthma, among others, are the result of unquantifiable spiritual suffering. As a result, and as the level of distress diminishes, these ailments will gradually disappear. Because the psychic energy, call it sexual or libidinal, contained by the process of repression, will cause an emotional cataclysm before exhausting itself in the formation of somatic manifestations and, in this process, may be the origin of many of the diseases that we today attribute, in exclusivity, to an organic origin.

Near the end of the journey, when few obstacles can impede that the facts can be accepted as presented without being disturbed by bastard interests, it is possible to manifest so risky statements, though not necessarily true. Looking back I can realize of, I would not speak of the errors, but of the impediments to see what was clearly shown to my observation. And it is difficult to meet two interests simultaneously: the social and the own.

I will explain: the beginning of the professional exercise coincides with the beginning of adult life that is characterized by the reversal of roles. The protagonism of those who come in search of a "solution" is promptly supplanted by the pride of who should be in the second plane. It is only at the end of a long journey when is possible to be close to anonymity, because, just as a concert is not possible to be enjoyed amid the hubbub, neither is advisable to look through a microscope with watery eyes.

THE END

# BIOGRAPHY

Born in Valencia de Don Juan (León) in 1941, Onésimo Fernández Rubio was graduated in Medicine and Surgery in 1968.

Medical specialty in Psychiatry, in1980, in Madrid.

Master on Psychoanalysis, in the Institute-Clinic "Peña Retama", in Hoyo de Manzanares (Madrid), under supervision of Dr. Jerónimo Molina Núñez.

Director of the Psychiatric Hospital "Santa Isabel", in León (Spain), from the year 1980 up to 1988.

I've been practicing the psychiatric specialty since 1968, under a basically psychoanalytic orientation, which began at the clinic "Peña Retama", at Hoyo de Manzanares (Madrid), a pioneer in Spain, as I believe, in the modality of therapeutic community. Subsequently I have exercised in others places, going by the direction of the Psychiatric Sanatorium "Santa Isabel", of Leon.

This publication, second of this genre -the previous one was titled "The Disease of Life"- is about the idea acquired on Psychiatry throughout my years of exercise and that can be summarized in the following: "The only remedy for not to suffer from the insults and the contempt that, erroneously, It is believed that they come from the own person, it is the precise knowledge through the steps that circumstances have imposed. In my opinion, both Psychology and Psychiatry -disciplines of impossible differentiation- have as their ultimate goal the implantation of the friendship within the inner world of the person".

In my opinion, both Psychology and Psychiatry - disciplines of impossible differentiation - have as their ultimate goal the implantation of friendship within the inner.

# AUTHORS' BOOKS

I practiced the psychiatric specialty since 1968, under a basically psychoanalytic orientation, which began at the clinic "Peña Retama", by Hoyo de Manzanares, a pioneer in Spain, as I believe, in the modality of therapeutic community. Subsequently I have exercised in various media, among then the direction of the Psychiatric Sanatorium "Santa Isabel", of Leon.

## THE DISEASE OF LIFE

From Coyanza´s Casino

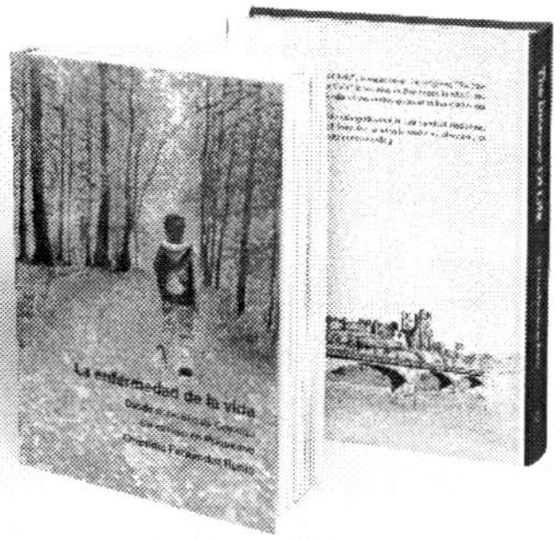


This work, "The Disease of Life", translation of the original, "La Enfermedad de La Vida" is an essay on Psychiatry in which the biographical details of the author go hand in hand with the medical studies. It aims to provide a simplification of this medical discipline, often presented from the academic world as abstruse, in order to his easier understanding.

## SUELTA HILO A LA COMETA

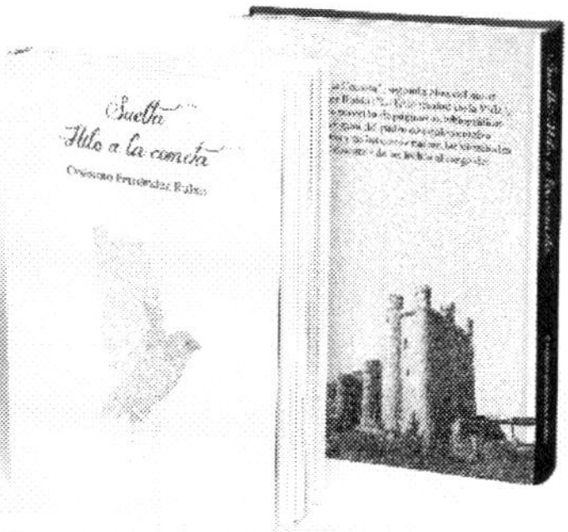


The second book of Onésimo Fernández Rubio, is the succession of autobiographical pages that revolve around the figure of the father with whom he establishes frequent colloquiums. In them the events lived throughout the dates are narrated to the position of the family business in the Casino of Valencia de Don Juan (Coyanza), León.

Learn more www.psiquiatriazaragoza.com

When the friendship of one wit himself has been lost or not established, it is the knowledge of oneself that enables the release of the unbearable experience of feeling "different" or "exiled." The attainment of "being oneself" is the highest desire of every person.

Made in United States
Troutdale, OR
11/03/2026

56845261R00127